TABLE OF CONTENTS

Top 20 Test Taking Tips

1. Carefully follow all the test registration procedures
2. Know the test directions, duration, topics, question types, how many questions
3. Setup a flexible study schedule at least 3-4 weeks before test day
4. Study during the time of day you are most alert, relaxed, and stress free
5. Maximize your learning style; visual learner use visual study aids, auditory learner use auditory study aids
6. Focus on your weakest knowledge base
7. Find a study partner to review with and help clarify questions
8. Practice, practice, practice
9. Get a good night's sleep; don't try to cram the night before the test
10. Eat a well balanced meal
11. Know the exact physical location of the testing site; drive the route to the site prior to test day
12. Bring a set of ear plugs; the testing center could be noisy
13. Wear comfortable, loose fitting, layered clothing to the testing center; prepare for it to be either cold or hot during the test
14. Bring at least 2 current forms of ID to the testing center
15. Arrive to the test early; be prepared to wait and be patient
16. Eliminate the obviously wrong answer choices, then guess the first remaining choice
17. Pace yourself; don't rush, but keep working and move on if you get stuck
18. Maintain a positive attitude even if the test is going poorly
19. Keep your first answer unless you are positive it is wrong
20. Check your work, don't make a careless mistake

Certified Specialist Pediatric Exam

Pediatric disorders

Pediatric diabetes

The center of the pediatric diabetes team should be the child, their parents and family because they will need to manage all the various aspects of the disease. The remainder of the team should include:

- Pediatric endocrinologist to provide medical care specific to diabetes
- Pediatrician who will care for the developmental and other medical needs of the child
- Registered dietitian specializing in pediatrics should also be included and would be responsible for educating the child and family on nutrition, and for tailoring a meal plan specific for that child
- Diabetes nurse educator who has experience and training in teaching the child and family about diabetes
- Pediatric social worker or child psychologist to assist with providing support for the family in integrating the disease into daily life
- Child life specialist who helps support the child through play
- School, babysitters, daycare or any other people involved in the child's life that provide direct care to the child
- Extended family such as grandparents, aunts, uncles, or close friends who may be responsible for caring for the child

Medical nutrition therapy

The goals for medical nutrition therapy include:

- Providing a meal plan that incorporates sound nutrition principles while taking into consideration a child's appetite, likes, dislikes and lifestyle.
- To maintain blood glucose levels as close to normal as possible to reduce the risk of developing short and long-term complications of diabetes.
- To maintaining normal growth and development and an appropriate body weight
- Maintain normal lipid values

- Assisting with the social and psychological aspects of diabetes
- To provide education to the family that takes into account learning ability, learning style, language, culture, ethnicity, and interest
- To review current research with the family so they are able to make appropriate decisions in treating diabetes

Meal plan design

The overall goals for determining a meal plan should be to provide healthy nutrition guidelines, encourage positive changes in behavior and to plan healthy meals and snacks. A meal plan should be highly individualized and should incorporate a child's appetite level and food preferences. The lifestyle of the child and family needs to be taken into account. The family should not be expected to change their lifestyle significantly to fit diabetes in, rather the family should be educated on how diabetes can be fit into the lifestyle they have, within reason. The entire family should be encouraged to follow the same guidelines as the child to help prevent the child from feeling isolated or abnormal. It should not be viewed that the child is following a "special diet". Healthy eating for everyone in the family should be stressed as a matter of health and wellness, not just because the child has diabetes. The child should be reassured that favorite foods and snacks will still be options.

Glycemic index

The glycemic index is a ranking system of how quickly a certain carbohydrate raises a person's blood glucose level. The glycemic index can be used as a marker of the general glucose response of a specific food. Foods with a low glycemic index are complex carbohydrates such as fruits and vegetables, and whole grains. These foods take longer to digest and produce a more stable blood glucose. Foods with a high glycemic index include refined carbohydrates such as white bread or potatoes. These foods are more rapidly digested causing a quicker rise in blood glucose levels. A moderate glycemic index includes foods such as candy, soft drinks, and some higher fat foods. The glycemic load may be a better tool for assessing a food's effect on blood glucose. It is the glycemic index multiplied by the amount of carbohydrate present in a food. This would more properly place foods based on blood glucose response and nutritional value. Candy bars would now be considered to have a high glycemic load instead of medium glycemic index.

Sweeteners

Sucrose

Sucrose can be a part of a healthy diet if the child consumes foods from all food groups and the sucrose is substituted for other carbohydrates rather than eaten in addition to the other carbohydrate sources. Often times, the source of sucrose is considered empty calories with limited nutritional value such as soft drinks or fruit drinks and should be consumed with caution. Other sucrose containing foods such as cake or cookies should be considered special treats and not routinely consumed. Other sweeteners such as corn syrup, honey, and molasses do not have any advantages over sucrose. Sugar alcohols such as sorbitol, mannitol or xylitol may have a lower glycemic response but are associated with gastrointestinal side effects if taken in large quantities. Fructose may cause a smaller rise in glucose levels; however, studies have shown fructose may have a negative effect on cholesterol and LDL levels.

Aspartame

The Nonnutritive sweetener aspartame is approved by the Food and Drug Administration (FDA) and has an Acceptable Daily Intake (ADI) recommendation. An ADI is the amount of food additive that can be safely ingested every day for a person's lifetime without adverse effects. A safety factor of 100 times above that number is included in the ADI. Aspartame contains 4 kcals per gram but is approximately 200 times sweeter than sucrose therefore provides minimal calories. Aspartame is not heat stable and may break down when exposed to prolonged high temperatures. It is widely used throughout the world and has not been associated with any adverse side effects. It does contain phenylalanine and its use should be restricted in people with phenylketonuria (PKU).

Saccharin and sucralose

The nonnutritive sweeteners acesulfame K, saccharin, and sucralose are also FDA approved. Acesulfame K has no calories and is not metabolized by the body. It is approximately 200 times sweeter than sucrose but is often blended with other sweeteners because it can have an aftertaste. It is heat stable and has been reported as safe.

Saccharin is up to 700 times as sweet as sucrose and contains no calories but can leave a bitter aftertaste at high concentrations. It is heat stable and is not metabolized by the body. Sucralose is the newest nonnutritive sweetener. It is up to 600 times sweeter than sucrose. It is made from sugar and does not affect blood glucose levels because it is not metabolized by the body. Sucralose is heat stable and can be used in baking.

Dyslipidemia

If dyslipidemia is identified on screening, treatment should commence with exercise and American Heart Association Step 2 diet. Fat restriction for children younger than 2 is not recommended due to the need for fat for brain development. Saturated fat should be restricted to less than 7% of total calories and cholesterol restricted to less than 200 mg per day. Trans fats should be restricted. Weight reduction may be indicated. Soluble fiber such as bran, oats, fruits and vegetables should be increased in the diet. Medication such as statins may be prescribed depending upon the LDL cholesterol level.

Vitamin and mineral supplements

Children with diabetes do not typically require multivitamin and mineral supplements if a balanced, nutritious diet is consumed and the child is growing appropriately. The nutritional adequacy of a child's diet tends to balance out over the course of a few days or a week. If a child's diet excludes certain food groups, supplementation would be indicated. If a specific micronutrient deficiency were identified, supplementation would also be appropriate. Chromium deficiency can lead to hyperglycemia, hypercholesterolemia, hypertriglyceridemia, and delayed growth. Chromium deficiency is rare in children and can be sometimes seen in the elderly or in patients receiving long-term parenteral nutrition. Routine chromium supplementation is not indicated unless a deficiency is documented. Magnesium deficiency can lead to insulin resistance and carbohydrate intolerance. Magnesium deficiency, however, is not normally seen in healthy children eating a balanced diet but can be seen in high-risk patients such as those in diabetic ketoacidosis or on diuretics.

Initial type 1 diabetes

Diagnosis

The child's weight and height for age and recent weight history should be obtained. The child should be plotted on the appropriate growth charts. Body Mass Index and ideal body weight should be calculated to as part of the nutritional assessment. The child's overall nutritional status should be assessed. A full diet history needs to be obtained including information regarding the family's schedule for both weekdays and weekends, and school or daycare information. The diet history should also include timing of meals. Activity level is important in order to calculate appropriate energy needs as well as insulin requirements.

Nutrition recommendations

Nutrition recommendations for a child with type 1 diabetes essentially encourage a healthy diet and are not different than recommendations for a child without diabetes. Calories should be calculated using the child's typical intake or the recommended dietary allowance (RDA) and should promote a normal growth pattern. Children who are newly diagnosed may require additional calories to regain lost weight. The carbohydrate allowance will vary based on assessment and the child's typical intake but should contribute no more than 55-60% of total calories. The protein allowance can be calculated at 10-20% of total calories or can be estimated using the RDA. The fat allowance should be individualized based on weight status, lipid levels, and family history. Less than 10% of total calories should be from saturated fat, and up to 30% of total calories can be from fat. Fiber is important to overall health. The American Academy of Pediatrics recommends 0.5 grams of fiber per kilogram of body weight with a maximum intake of 35 grams. Another method to estimate fiber requirements is age plus 5 grams for children ages 2-20.

Lipid levels

Type 1 diabetes increases the risk for cardiovascular disease; however, blood glucose control may also directly affect lipid levels. Children should not be screened for dyslipidemia until normal glucose levels are achieved. If tested at diagnosis, lipid levels will likely be elevated related to hyperglycemia. Once glucose levels are controlled, children with a family history of heart disease before age 55 or with a family history of total cholesterol level greater than 240 mg/dl should be screened at diagnosis then every 5 years after puberty if lipid levels are normal. For children without any significant family history, screening can begin at puberty. For children with type 2 diabetes, lipids should be screened at diagnosis then every 2 years. Lipid goals should be less than 100 mg/dl for LDL cholesterol, greater than 35 mg/dl for HDL cholesterol and triglycerides less than 150 mg/dl.

Laboratory data

Blood glucose levels should be noted and followed as diabetes comes under control. A chromium test is not indicated, as deficiency is rare and unlikely. A glucose tolerance test is not indicated if the diagnosis has already been made and may actually cause harm if conducted. Urine ketones would be expected given the new diagnosis of type 1 diabetes and will not provide helpful information for initial evaluation. Lipid levels will likely be elevated related to hyperglycemia at diagnosis and will not be useful for initial evaluation. A glycosylated hemoglobin (HgbA1C) does not need to be checked at diagnosis, as an elevated level will only reflect the untreated diabetes prior to diagnosis. A blood urea nitrogen (BUN) would not provide useful information on renal status, as it will reflect hydration status at time of diagnosis.   The goal for fasting blood glucose levels for children less than 6 is 100-180 mg/dl, for children 6-12 90-180 mg/dl, and for age 12 and older 90-150 mg/dl.

Initial meal plan and nutrition counseling

The parent and child should begin to keep a food record for every meal, snack and beverage and timing to help determine the amount of food needed based on appetite. The food record should also include insulin and blood glucose levels. Appetite can be elevated at the time of diagnosis due to loss of sugar in the urine. Adequate food should be provided to help discourage the child from associating hunger and food limitations with diabetes. The initial meal plan should try to include the amount of food the child likes to eat if possible. A range of food choices should be offered in order to provide additional food if the child desires. The meal plan may need fine tuning every 2-3 weeks after initial diagnosis as appetite and weight return to normal. Initial counseling should be geared to the child and family's readiness to learn, ability to learn and interest. General guidelines should be provided regarding types of food and carbohydrates, the importance of regular and consistent meals and snacks, timing of meals and portion sizes. Initial survival skills use this goal and this may require 2-4 hours of education.

Positive encouragement

A positive relationship is essential in working with a child with diabetes. The child should be included in the interview and meal planning. The child should be reassured that favorite foods can still be a part of their meals. Negative words should be avoided such as restrict, do not, and never to try to prevent any negative connotations. The adolescent child should initially be interviewed separately then together with the parents to try to begin self-management training. Encourage the parents to listen carefully to their child when requesting special food so this may be worked into the meal plan when possible. The parents should try to avoid saying no all the time and not be viewed as the food police. Parents and caregivers need to be educated not to give less food based on high blood glucose levels as this may lead to hypoglycemia.

Weight control and disordered eating

As children grow and mature into adolescents, weight issues can often arise. Occasionally weight gain will precede a gain in height. The weight should be stabilized to allow the height to proportionately fit the child's weight. A calorie restricted diet is not recommended in many cases because of possible adverse effects on growth and development. Increasing activity levels is a good alternative to help with weight control. Some adolescents with weight issues may choose to omit insulin shots to cause weight loss. This is a dangerous habit and can lead to disordered eating. Signs that an adolescent may be skipping insulin doses are a weight change of 10 or more pounds, elevated glycosylated hemoglobin level, uncontrolled diabetes, multiple episodes of diabetic ketoacidosis (DKA), or resistance to increasing insulin regimen. The child may also show signs of disordered eating such as excessive worries about weight or excessive exercise. An education plan should be implemented by an RD or Certified Diabetes Educator (CDE) about the dangers of disordered eating with diabetes.

Carbohydrate counting

Carbohydrate counting is a system used that allows for more flexibility in meal planning, timing of meals, portion sizes and types of food consumed. Carbohydrate intake is coordinated with the type of insulin provided and resulting blood glucose levels. The endocrinologist identifies target blood glucose levels then an insulin to carbohydrate ratio is determined. Generally a short acting insulin is used such as humalog or novolog. Typically, 1 unit of short acting insulin covers 10-15 grams of carbohydrate but this varies based on the individual's age, activity level and insulin requirements. A basic knowledge of carbohydrate containing foods, the effect of carbohydrate on blood glucose, and portion control is required for this system to be effective. Reading food labels is important and books are commercially available that provide carbohydrate information to assist with meal planning.

Insulin types and therapy

Very rapid acting insulin types include humalog and novolog. The onset of action is 10-30 minutes with a peak of 30 minutes to 3 hours. The duration of very rapid acting insulin is 3-5 hours. Lispro is also a rapid acting insulin with an onset less than 15 minutes, a peak of 0.5-1.5 hours and a duration of 2-4 hours. Rapid acting insulin is known as regular insulin. Its onset is 30 minutes with a peak of 1-5 hours. The duration of rapid acting is 8 hours. Intermediate acting insulin types include NPH and lente. The onset of this type of insulin is 1-4 hours with a peak of 4-15 hours for NPH and 4-12 hours for lente. The duration is 14-26 hours for NPH and 16-26 hours for lente. Long acting insulin types include ultralente and lantus. The onset of ultralente is 4-6 hours with a peak of 8-30 hours and a duration of 24-36 hours. For lantus, the onset is 1-2 hours with a duration of 24 hours. There is no peak action for lantus.

<u>Lantus</u>
Lantus (glargine) is an excellent choice for many children and adolescents because it offers the flexibility that an insulin pump would provide without needing the equipment associated with using the pump. Lantus is given once per day by injection in the evening or at bedtime. Occasionally the dose is split between two doses given 12 hours apart. A rapid

acting insulin is given when carbohydrates are consumed or if blood glucose levels need to be reduced. The number of shots required per day may be as high as 6. Lantus is often trialed prior to starting pump therapy to make sure the child and family have acquired the necessary skills for self-management. These skills include advanced carbohydrate counting, insulin to carbohydrate ratios, ability to correct or adjust insulin doses based on blood glucose levels and appropriate math skills. Typical daily dosing for basal insulin requirements using Lantus is approximately 0.5-1.5 units per kg body weight though adolescents may need up to 3 units per kg.

Therapy

Conventional insulin therapy refers to 1-2 injections per day of intermediate acting insulin or long acting insulin. A small amount of short acting insulin is sometimes included in this regimen. Intensive insulin therapy refers to 4 or more injections per day of short acting insulin combined with either intermediate or long acting insulin. CSII pump therapy can also be used in conjunction with intensive therapy. CSII pump therapy is an option for a pediatric patient that has greatly improved blood glucose control, improved linear growth and helps prevent diabetic ketoacidosis. Pump therapy provides fast acting insulin and is delivered in small boluses throughout the day to cover meals, snacks and elevated blood glucose levels.

Meal planning considerations

Because conventional insulin therapy uses intermediate or long acting insulin, the peak action must be taken into account. Children should eat a snack between each meal and before bed to prevent hypoglycemia. For young children, the snack should consist of 15-20 grams of carbohydrate and 20-30 grams for adolescents. Exercise and physical activity should also be taken into account and a larger snack provided for these occasions. The snack should contain 20-30 grams of carbohydrate and 1-2 ounces of protein to help keep blood glucose levels stable. The main challenge with this type of insulin therapy is consistent meals and carbohydrate intake. The amount of carbohydrate should remain relatively consistent from meal to meal and snack to snack. This would typically be 30-45 grams carbohydrate per meal for children age 5 or less, 45-60 grams for children ages 5-12 and 45-75 grams for children older than 12.

Diabetes management

Infants and toddlers pose a unique challenge for diabetes management because of irregular or unpredictable eating patterns. Also, young children are not able to understand the need for injections that may make insulin therapy even more difficult. The main goal is avoiding hypoglycemia, as this is dangerous for developing brains. For elementary age children, adjusting to the school schedule can be difficult. Challenges can include unpredictable activity levels, feelings of being different and getting the child more involved in self-management. At this age, the child should have a basic understanding of diabetes and the long-term complications that may develop if diabetes is not properly managed. The adolescent faces many challenges as well including trying to fit in with their peers, taking more responsibility for self-management, and keeping blood glucose levels under control during periods of growth. Adolescents often have to work through feelings of anger regarding diabetes. As the adolescent approaches the late teen years, he/she should be able to independently self manage diabetes care.

Type 2 diabetes

Over the last 10-15 years, the incidence of type 2 diabetes in children is rising at an alarming rate and if the rate continues to rise, this will present significant heath care challenges. This significant increase is positively correlated with the rise in obesity in children. A high number of cases occur in ethnic minorities including Mexican-American, African-American, Asian- American and Native American. Children with a body mass index greater than 85, a weight greater than 120% of ideal, a positive family history of diabetes and signs of insulin resistance such as high blood pressure or hyperlipidemia should be screened for type 2 diabetes. Nutrition counseling should be initiated to help the child or adolescent achieve and maintain a healthy body weight. Increasing physical activity is a priority as well. Often times, medication such as metformin or even insulin are started. In addition, children who are at risk for developing type 2 diabetes should also receive intervention for diet and exercise.

<u>Management</u>

Regular exercise provides many benefits to those with diabetes such as maintaining or improving glucose levels, improving lipid levels and weight control. In children, regular aerobic exercise can help to prevent obesity and can help to keep the heart healthy. A minimum of 30-60 minutes per day is a realistic goal. Blood glucose levels should be monitored before, during and after exercise. Exercise should not occur with blood glucose levels less than 120 mg/dl, greater than 240 mg/dl with ketones present or with blood glucose greater than 400 mg/dl. Caution must be taken to prevent hypoglycemia from occurring during exercise. A snack can be taken prior to exercise or if the exercise routine is consistent from day to day, the child's insulin can be adjusted accordingly. The size of the snack will depend upon how long the exercise will last and how intense the workout is. A rule of thumb is 10-15 grams of carbohydrate for each hour of additional activity. Adding a protein source is also a good idea to prevent hypoglycemia after the exercise has stopped.

Hypoglycemia

Hypoglycemia is commonly caused by skipping or delaying a meal or snack or too little food eaten is relation to insulin prescribed. The symptoms of hypoglycemia can include shakiness, headache, hunger, sweating, and palpitations. If untreated, hypoglycemia can lead to confusion, extreme fatigue, lethargy, seizures and unconsciousness. A blood glucose level less than 70 mg/dl should be treated. It is important to note that each person's response to hypoglycemia is different as is the blood glucose level that symptoms occur. To treat hypoglycemia, a readily available source of sugar such as glucose tablets, juice, sugar, soda, or lifesavers should be given. For children age 5 and younger, 5-10 grams of carbohydrate is recommended. For children ages 6-10, 10-15 grams is recommended and for children older than 10, 15-20 grams of carbohydrate should be given. In extreme cases, glucagons should be administered.

<u>Treatment</u>

First and foremost, insulin should never be omitted. The dose may need to be reduced under physician guidance but insulin should still be given. If the child has persistent vomiting, diarrhea, or fever, the parents should contact the child's physician for assistance. This type of illness can quickly lead to dehydration and diabetic ketoacidosis.

The child's blood glucose and urine ketones should be monitored every 3-4 hours to watch for this. If the child is not able to maintain their normal meal pattern, sugar containing liquids such as juice, soda, sports drinks, regular Jell-O, or Popsicles should be substituted in order to provide energy for the body. If the blood glucose level is >120-150, sugar-free drinks can be given.

Diabetic ketoacidosis

The diabetes care team will help to determine how often blood glucose levels should be monitored. There is no set number of times per day that blood glucose levels should be checked but for those receiving insulin, generally need to check at least 3-4 times per day. The best way to know if diabetes is being effectively managed and blood glucoses are in the target range is to monitor frequently. During illness, the frequency would increase. Illness increases the risk of developing diabetic ketoacidosis (DKA), which is a state of metabolic disarray occurring in patients with type 1 diabetes due to inadequate insulin and excessive stress hormone response. DKA can occur when blood glucose levels are greater than 200 mg/dl, ketones are present in the urine or blood, and an acidosis is present. This is a very serious consequence that requires hospitalization and can lead to cardiac issues, severe acidosis, hypokalemia, cerebral edema and death if untreated.

Pre-term infants

Infants born prematurely are born before the 37th week of gestation. Preterm infants are classified according to their birth weight. Low birth weight (LBW) infants are less than 2 kg, very low birth weight (VLBW) infants are less than 1.5 kg, and extremely low birth weight (ELBW) infants are less that 1 kg. Preterm infants can be further classified according to their weight for gestational age. A small for gestational age infant (SGA) has a birth weight less than the 10%, appropriate for gestational age (AGA) has a birth weight greater than the 10% and less than the 90%, while large for gestational age (LGA) has a birth weight greater than the 90%.

Parenteral nutrition

Ideally, parenteral nutrition (PN) including amino acids should be started within 24 hours of life. Studies have shown benefits to starting PN within a few hours of birth. Multiple studies have shown that early administration of amino acids promotes positive nitrogen balance and stimulates protein synthesis. Preterm infants lose protein at a very rapid rate and it can be very difficult to replete protein stores. Early amino acids administration also helps to improve blood glucose levels, which in turn will allow for greater caloric intake with dextrose. PN is indicated for low birth weight infants because the gastrointestinal tract is not yet ready to assume full enteral nutrition so soon after birth. In addition, preterm infants are at risk for necrotizing enterocolitis and enteral nutrition must be initiated slowly. The overall goal for early PN administration is to reduce catabolism, provide nutrients and encourage growth until enteral feedings can be provided at a level to support the necessary growth.

Enteral nutrition

Infants born prematurely have not had enough time for full gastrointestinal (GI) development. The earlier the infant is born and the lower the birth weight, the greater the risk the infant would have for developing necrotizing enterocolitis (NEC). Immature GI tracts will also have limited gastric emptying. Respiratory distress may delay enteral nutrition due to the risk for aspiration. Critically ill preterm infants with cardiac instability, severe acidosis, hypotension or hypoxemia will not be fed enterally until their condition improves. An infant that develops a patent ductus arteriosus (PDA) requiring treatment with indocin will most likely not receive enteral nutrition because of the concern for decreased blood perfusion in the gut. Preterm infants receiving an exchange transfusion for hyperbilirubinemia will not be fed enterally due the risk for NEC. Finally, infants with sepsis will not initially receive enteral nutrition due to concerns with decreased gut perfusion and possible NEC.

Trophic feedings

Trophic feedings are defined as small volume feedings delivered at a low rate. Because preterm infants are at risk for developing necrotizing enterocolitis (NEC), enteral feedings must be initiated and advanced slowly and cautiously. Trophic feedings are considered to be nonnutritive and used more for gut stimulation. Breast milk or preterm formula can be used although breast milk is preferred. The benefits to trophic feedings are many and include improved feeding tolerance, reaching full enteral feedings quicker, promoting intestinal maturation, stimulating gut hormones, and decreasing intestinal transit time allowing for better nutrient absorption. Other clinical benefits include improved bilirubin and less phototherapy requirements, reducing the risk of cholestasis, improved alkaline phosphatase levels and improved bone mineralization. Overall length of hospital stay may be shorter.

Iron supplementation

Preterm infants are at risk for a variety of vitamin and mineral deficiencies due to decreased stores at birth, inadequate intake or altered metabolism. Iron deficiency is possible because major iron deposition occurs during the third trimester of pregnancy so infants born prematurely are born with limited stores. Blood loss, gestational age, growth rate and initial hemoglobin level will affect iron status. Infants that receive PN for a prolonged period will be at further risk. Preterm infants require 2-4 mg/kg and up to 6 mg/kg if erythropoietin therapy is given. Iron requirements of 2 mg/kg can be met with an iron fortified preterm formula fed at 120 kcal/kg. If the baby receives breast milk, iron supplementation can be provided after the infant reaches full enteral feedings or at one month of age. Some human milk fortifiers contain a small amount of iron.

Vitamin A and E

Vitamin E has been studied as a possible treatment to prevent retinopathy of prematurity, bronchopulmonary dysplasia (BPD), or intraventricular hemorrhage, however, studies have not demonstrated success therefore pharmacological doses of vitamin E are not recommended. Vitamin A supplementation has been studied as a possible treatment for preventing BPD. Some benefits have been shown, however, rates of BPD vary greatly between NICU's and supplements must be given intramuscularly. The risks and benefits must be weighed carefully for each NICU, as there are many other treatment options available to help prevent BPD.

Osteopenia of prematurity

Osteopenia of prematurity is poor bone mineralization as a result of insufficient calcium and phosphorus intake. Preterm infants are at risk for osteopenia for many reasons. Major calcium deposition in bones occurs during the third trimester of pregnancy therefore, infants born prematurely do not receive this deposition. Other risk factors include prolonged PN because it is difficult to meet calcium and phosphorus requirements due to solubility issues. Unfortified breast milk and the use of standard term formula increase the risk because calcium and phosphorus content is inadequate. The use of soy formula also increases the risk due to phytates that are present in the formula binding with phosphorus making it unavailable. Certain medications such as Lasix increase the risk because it increases urinary calcium excretion. Enteral requirements for calcium are 120-230 mg/kg and 60-140 mg/kg for phosphorus. Vitamin D requirements are 150-400 units per day. Preterm infants receiving preterm formula or fortified breast m ilk should be able to meet requirements for bone development.

Assessing growth

Infants should be weighed at approximately the same time every day and on the same scale for more accuracy. Daily weights are used for a number of reasons including measuring growth and monitoring fluid status. Initial weight loss of up to 15% can be expected in preterm infants; however, birth weight should be regained by 2 weeks of life. Weight is assessed by monitoring for trends over several days or a week. Weights should be plotted on the appropriate growth chart to determine the adequacy of growth and caloric intake. Length should be measured once per week, ideally on a recumbent length board. The same clinician should measure length each week if possible for consistency. Expected length gains are 0.8- 1.1 cm per week. Head circumference should be measured weekly for growth purposes and plotted on the appropriate growth chart. Appropriate gain would be 0.5-0.8 cm per week.

Fluid, dextrose, amino acids, and lipids

Parenteral nutrition (PN) should be initiated within 24 hours of birth. Ideally, PN would be started within hours of birth. Fluids can generally be provided at 60-140 cc/kg per day then gradually increased. Glucose requirements initially are 4-8 mg/kg/minute to maintain normal blood glucose levels. Glucose concentration can be increased by 2 mg/kg/minute (or by approximately 2.5% dextrose) to a maximum of 12-15 mg/kg/minute. Amino acids can be safely started at 1-2 grams/kg and can be advanced by 0.5-1 gram/kg to a goal of 3-3.8 grams/kg. Lipids can be started on the first day of life. Essential fatty acid deficiency can develop in as little as two days without a lipid source as preterm infants have very limited stores. Lipids can be safely initiated at 0.5-1 gram/kg and advanced by 0.5-1 gram/kg to a goal of 3 grams/kg.

Laboratory data

Initial laboratory data in a preterm infant includes:

- Sodium, potassium, chloride
- Blood urea nitrogen (BUN), creatinine
- Blood glucose
- Calcium, phosphorus, magnesium
- Triglycerides
- Albumin and total protein
- Liver function tests including alkaline phosphatase
- Total and direct bilirubin
- Hemoglobin, hematocrit and platelets
- Urine glucose and ketones

The above-mentioned labs should be checked daily until stable or if adjustments are made in the PN solution.

Nutritional risk factors

Preterm infants have many nutritional risk factors. Calorie and protein requirements are elevated compared to term infants because of the rapid growth and tissue development that occurs. The stress of being in the NICU and complications of prematurity also adds risk. Preterm infants have difficulty with temperature regulation, which increases caloric requirements. Preterm infants also have varying degrees of organ function depending upon gestational age. The GI tract is immature. Renal function is also immature and can receive added stress due to many reasons including medications. Nutrient stores are sub optimal because of prematurity. Preterm infants do not develop the suck/swallow/breathe reflex until 32-34 weeks gestation therefore enteral nutrition cannot be given by mouth.

Preterm infant discharge

Prior to a discharge to home, the preterm infant needs to be able to take all feedings safely by mouth and be able to consistently gain approximately 30 grams per day. In certain cases, the discharge plan may include nasogastric or gastrostomy feedings. The infant should be receiving the appropriate transitional formula for discharge. If the infant is breast feeding, consistent weight gain is important as well as ability to effectively nurse. Whatever the feeding plan is, the parents should be fully educated on the plan and should be encouraged to room in with the baby before discharge to be comfortable. The infant should be evaluated for the WIC program if appropriate. Referral to NICU follow-up program is essential. Preterm infants will continue to be at risk for nutritional deficiencies after discharge. Infants that are particularly at risk include birth weight less than 1.5 kg, small for gestational age infants, infants with a history of poor weight gain and a history of poor feeding. Infants with preterm complications such as NEC, BPD and osteopenia are also at continued risk.

Bronchopulmonary dysplasia

Bronchopulmonary dysplasia (BPD) is a type of chronic lung disease that mainly affects premature infants and is caused by high oxygen concentrations and prolonged mechanical ventilation. Preterm infants with abnormal chest X-rays and who require supplemental oxygen on the 28th day are considered to have BPD. Infants with BPD generally have an elevated basal metabolic rate and increased work on breathing. Both of these increase caloric requirements and impact growth if the additional caloric needs are not met. Growth failure is common in infants with BPD and catch up growth is often required. In order for growth to occur, adequate calories must be consumed and adequate oxygenation needs to be delivered. This especially needs to happen at night during sleep. Studies have shown that improved growth can occur during sleep in infants with BPD. Oxygen saturation levels should be greater than 92%.

Nutritional status
Infants with BPD may experience higher rates of illness, which will adversely affect caloric intake and will impact nutritional status. Many infants have elevated respiratory rates, which can affect the infant's ability to feed efficiently and effectively. This can also alter the suck/swallow/breathe reflex and may cause the infant to tire easily. BPD often requires the use of diuretics for management and may also require a fluid and sodium restriction. A fluid restriction usually requires the use of a concentrated formula in order to provide

appropriate caloric intake for growth. Certain diuretics increase urinary calcium excretion and place the infant at risk for osteopenia. Infants with BPD often require prolonged ventilation in the neonatal period using an endotracheal tube. This can cause oral aversion and affect the infant's suck/swallow/breathe reflex. Gastroesophageal reflux is also common following prolonged intubation.

Caloric requirements

Calorie requirements for infants with BPD can be up to 50% higher than for healthy infants. This is roughly equivalent to 50% above the RDA or 120-150 kcal/kg for enteral requirements. Some infants may require even more calories for catch up growth to occur. As lung function improves, caloric requirements may gradually decrease. Infants with BPD often require a fluid restriction or may be unable to take adequate formula volume to meet caloric requirements. Concentrating the formula is an option. Formulas can be concentrated to 24-30 kcal/ounce. As the concentration increases, the osmolality and renal solute load also increases and may affect tolerance. The osmolality of the formula should be less than 400 mOsm/liter. A mix of preterm formula, standard formula concentrate or modular products such as polycose or microlipid can be used to achieve desired concentration. The infant should meet basic protein, vitamin and mineral requirements while maintaining an appropriate nutrient distribution.

Gastroesophageal reflux

Gastroesophageal reflux (GER) is the regurgitation of gastric contents into the esophagus. This is a painful condition. Infants with GER will often arch their backs, turn away from the nipple, cry frequently and spit up while experiencing symptoms. Infants with GER are at risk for failure to thrive, aspiration and inflammation of the esophagus. Treatment includes proper positioning into the upright position and small, frequent feedings to reduce volume consumed. A concentrated formula may be needed to meet caloric requirements. Medications such as antacids, proton pump inhibitors, H2 receptor antagonists and prokinetic agents are often initiated. Rice cereal is often used for treating GER, however, studies have not effectively documented its benefit. Rice cereal may help to reduce the number of times GER is experiences or may reduce crying. It also can increase the risk for malabsorption of complex carbohydrates that the infant is not yet developmentally ready to digest and reduces the nutrient composition of the formula.

Growth

Typical growth patterns

Birth and age 2 and ages 3-6

Growth patterns are individual and are influenced in part by genetics. Typical growth patterns from birth to age 2 include doubling of birth weight by 5 months and tripling birth weight by 1 year. The brain doubles its weight by age 1 and head circumference will increase approximately 10 cm in the first year. Length will increase approximately 12 cm between age 1 and 2. Preschool age children (ages 3-6) have a growth pattern that slows down until around age 4-5. At this time, the child will grow 6-8 cm annually and will gain 2-4 kg per year. Brain weight will triple by age 6.

Ages 7-10 and 11-18

During middle childhood (ages 7-10), growth continues. An increase of 5-6 cm and a weight gain of approximately 2 kg per year can be expected. Girls tend to grow slightly quicker than boys during this period. At the age of 10, girls will be about 1 cm taller than boys and tend to be bigger when adolescence starts. During the adolescent period, the first growth spurt for girls will occur around age 11-14. Boys tend to hit their growth spurts approximately 2 years after girls and this growth spurt is longer in duration with larger gains. Boys can gain 9.5-10.5 cm per year in height and girls can gain 8.5-9 cm per year. Girls tend to add more body fat while boys add more muscle mass. Growth is usually completed around age 16-18 for girls and 18-20 for boys.

2 weight percentiles

If a former preterm infant has not grown satisfactorily and has crossed 2 weight percentiles, a full nutrition assessment should be completed. Possible nutrition interventions may include a general review of overall weight history with clear and definitive goals for expected growth in the following months. Changes in formula concentration or diet may be indicated especially if inappropriate foods are being provided at the expense of nutritionally dense formula. Counseling or review of proper formula preparation and proper introduction to solids may be required. Referral to a feeding specialist such as a pediatric occupational therapist or speech language pathologist may be indicated if feeding difficulties are present. Referral to an early intervention program or the WIC program may also be appropriate.

Catch up growth

Catch up growth is an improvement in the growth rate after a period of growth failure. Infants who were born small for gestational age (SGA) will have a slower rate of catch up growth compared to infants born appropriate for gestational age (AGA). Head circumference is generally the first parameter to catch up and will occur sometime between 3-8 months with appropriate nutrition. Weight will catch up next followed by length. Most low birth weight infants will catch up by age 2-3 but some studies have shown that this may occur in the adolescent years as well. The ability to catch up is influenced by many factors including parental size and the presence of ongoing complications such as bronchopulmonary dysplasia. The child's growth curve should be followed closely with the goal of following his or her own growth curve, or paralleling the growth curve is growing below the 5 percentile.

Growth charts

The Lubchenco growth chart is a chart that uses intra uterine growth data and allows the plotting of weight, length, and head circumference from 24-42 weeks gestation. The data from this chart was obtained from infants born at high altitudes, which can have an adverse effect on growth. The Babson Benda chart uses intra-uterine and postnatal data collected throughout the first year of life but is limited by its small sample size. Less than 50 infants were born at a gestational age of less than 30 weeks. The data is from 1959-1963 and may not be representative of premature babies born today given the advances in perinatal and neonatal care. The Fenton growth charts are considered to be an updated version of the Babson Benda charts. It is a meta- analysis of reference studies to utilize newer data sets. Data can be plotted beginning at 22 weeks gestation.

Corrected age

Corrected age is adjusting an infant's current age for prematurity. This is also called post-conceptual age. To calculate this, you take the infant's chronological age minus the number of weeks or months the infant was premature. Using corrected age is helpful when plotting children on NCHS growth charts and should be used until the child is 18-36 months. While in the NICU, a preterm infant should average approximately 15-20 grams/kg of weight gain per day. Once the infant reaches a weight of 1.8 kg or reaches post conceptual age of 37 weeks, weight gain should be at least 20 grams per day from term to 3 months. As the infant gets older, the minimum weight gain is 15 grams/day for ages 3-6 months, 10 grams per day for ages 6-9 months, 6 grams per day for ages 9-12 months. This is the minimum weight gain and a higher rate may be expected. The main goal is a consistent growth pattern paralleling the established curve.

Waterlow and Gomez criteria

The Waterlow criteria evaluates the degree of stunting by determining the height for age percentile as a marker of chronic malnutrition. It evaluates the degree of wasting by determining the weight for height percentile as a marker for acute malnutrition. The categories are divided into normal, mild, moderate, or severe. The Gomez criterion evaluates weight for age but does not consider height or length. This criterion categorizes based on the degree of under nutrition. It does not take into account that a child of shorter height may have an appropriate weight for height and not actually be underweight. These categories are also divided into normal, mild, moderate, and severe degrees.

Growth failure

Medical history
The medical history of the child should include the birth history including APGAR scores, complications at delivery, prenatal care, gestational age at birth and birth weight, length and head circumference. The growth history should be reviewed ideally since birth. Information regarding when developmental milestones were attained should be documented. The child's history of acute or chronic illnesses along with any hospitalizations should be reviewed. A full mediation list should be obtained to look for any drug nutrient interactions or side effects of medications. A detailed family history is also important including history or psychiatric or psychological illness, substance abuse or eating disorders. Any genetic or in- born errors of metabolism or other metabolic disorders should be investigated as well as any chronic illnesses in the family. Information on parental height is useful as is the developmental and growth history of the child's siblings.

Clinical exam

The physical exam is generally done by a physician or nurse although the RD can also do a visual assessment observing for any signs of nutrient deficiency, easting and general appearance. The clinical exam should include screening for clinical signs of malnutrition, presence of GI issues such as nausea or vomiting, stool characteristics (frequency, color, amount, consistency, odor). The overall general condition of the child including signs of neglect or abuse, overall cleanliness and the condition of the mouth and teeth if present should be evaluated. Accurate height or length, weight and head circumference should be obtained and plotted on NCHS growth charts that ideally should include other points of reference for growth parameters. An assessment of development, fine and gross motor skills should be completed as well as documentation of any dysmorphic features.

Social history

A thorough social history is important when assessing a child with growth failure. The social situation should be evaluated including where the child lives, marital issues, domestic violence, financial issues and overall socioeconomic status. The parent or caregiver should be evaluated for maturity, mental stability, presence of significant stressors, availability of support system and how the problem is being viewed. Any history of neglect or abuse either to the child being assessed or any siblings should be documented. Any other caregivers such as babysitters, daycare providers or relatives should be identified. Information about the use of food stamps, WIC or any public assistance should be obtained. Parental and family views on eating and eating habits are important to consider as well as parental state of mind such as depression or lower learning ability.

Nutrition and feeding history

A thorough nutrition and feeding history should be obtained in the assessment of a child with growth failure. A 24-hour recall should be taken and if possible, 3-5 day food record should be recorded by the parent or caregiver. If the child is breastfeeding, a thorough assessment including techniques, length and frequency of nursing sessions should be obtained. Formula history should be obtained including information on formula preparation, frequency of feeding, tolerance, etc. For children who are eating solid food, the age when solids were introduced should be noted along with any food allergies or intolerances, and any diet restrictions. Information on timing of meals and snacks, who prepares and serves the meals, the location and how long the meal lasts should be noted. Quantities of juice, sweetened beverages, milk, and water taken each day should be obtained. The child's ability to feed self, information of behavior at meals and types of activities going on around the child when eating should be evaluated. The use of rewards or punishment related to food and eating should be noted.

Laboratory data

Growth failure in many cases is related to poor nutrition or social factors. A full laboratory panel as listed below is not always warranted and should be evaluated on a case-by-case basis. The following may be helpful:

- Lead screening
- Screening for iron deficiency anemia by checking hemoglobin and hematocrit. If these are low, full iron studies can be completed including iron, iron binding capacity, ferritin, and reticulocyte count.
- Urinalysis to include specific gravity and pH
- Serum sodium, potassium, chloride and glucose
- Albumin and prealbumin
- Renal function including BUN and creatinine
- Alkaline phosphatase level to check for the presence of rickets (if elevated) or for zinc deficiency (if low)
- If abnormal bowel habits are present, check stool studies to look for ova and parasites, occult blood, pH and reducing substances to help rule out malabsorption
- Sweat test for Cystic Fibrosis
- Tuberculosis test

Observing the parent or caregiver interaction

An observation of the interaction between the child and the parent or caregiver especially during mealtime is important. The overall bonding of the child in terms of physical contact, loving interaction, real warmth and affection, and response to the child's cues should be assessed. The expectations of the parent or caregiver should be evaluated for appropriateness. For instance, a child just over a year old cannot be expected to completely feed him or herself the entire meal without requiring assistance. The tolerance and stress level of the parent or caregiver should be assessed as well. Perhaps the parent gets angry about spilled food or soiled clothing at meal times.

Other factors

During the first 2 months of life, the goal is for the infant to reach a state of homeostasis. This means forming rhythms between being asleep and awake, feeding and elimination. It is also learning how to get his or her needs met by crying or other cues. A child who does not have his or her needs met will have a disordered homeostasis. The attachment phase occurs between 2 and 6 months of age when increased interaction occurs. Attachment disorder can occur if the infant continually receives negative interaction with the parent or caregiver. Common signs in this phase that a disorder is present include nausea, vomiting or diarrhea and poor weight gain. The third phase is separation and individualization that occurs between 6months and 3 years. This involves the child's quest for autonomy and the need for the parent to allow this to happen. Conflicts that can arise here include force feeding but the parent, refusal to sit down and eat by the child or aversion to multiple foods or textures.

Nutrition intervention

Three goals that should be accomplished with nutrition intervention include attaining the appropriate growth rate to reach an acceptable weight for length or height, ensuring that sufficient micro- and macro- nutrients are provided to meet requirements for growth, and detailed nutrition education with specific action steps for the parent or caregiver with a plan individually tailored to the child. There are a number of ways that calorie and protein needs can be calculated. These methods include using the RDA for calories as a base then adding 20-30% more for catch up growth, using the basal metabolic rate then adding activity factors, or using the Schofield equation that is reportedly similar to using resting energy requirements and using this number in the catch up growth equation instead of RDA. One method of calculating for catch up growth involves determining the RDA for age and determining the ideal weight at the 50% for the child's height. The equation is: (RDA calories for age X ideal weight for height in kg) divided by actual weight.

Interventions for a formula fed infant

Each plan for intervention needs to be tailored to the individual infant. Calorie and protein needs for catch up growth should be calculated and daily fluid requirements should be evaluated. Infants less than one year should not be consuming any soda or sweetened beverages and juice should be limited to 4 ounces per day for infants over 6 months. Water

- 28 -

should not be provided. Infant formula should be the main beverage for the infant. The caloric concentration of formula can be gradually increased up to 24-27 kcal/ounce by concentration. If the caloric density needs to increase further to meet caloric requirements, the use of modular products such as vegetable oil or polycose can be added up to 30 kcal/ounce. The percentage of fat in the formula should not exceed 55% as this may affect gastric emptying and affect tolerance. Close monitoring of tolerance for a calorically dense formula is required.

Interventions for a breastfed infant

For a breastfed infant, breastfeeding can continue, however, the use of supplemental bottles may need to be considered using higher calorie breast milk or formula. Infant formula powder or modular products can be added to breast milk to increase the caloric density. If the mom is averse to introducing a bottle, a supplemental nursing system (SNS) can be trialed. A bottle containing higher calorie breast milk or formula is connected to tubing that is then taped to the mom's breast. The tube is placed in the infant's mouth while he or she is breastfeeding so while nursing, the higher calorie formulation is also being provided. The use of hind milk, which is higher in fat and calories than foremilk, can also be helpful in increasing calorie intake. Consultation with a certified lactation specialist is recommended.

Interventions for a toddler

Interventions for a toddler with growth failure should include both dietary and behavior modifications. There are many dietary interventions available. Replacing water, juice or soda with whole milk mixed with instant breakfast powder or commercial supplements is one intervention. Adding calories to food such as with butter, oil, eggs, cream cheese, cheese, or powdered milk is another option. Serving foods with added sauces, salad dressing or gravies is another option. Offer foods that are not difficult to chew or swallow. Behavior modifications include setting a regular feeding schedule to include 3 meals and 3 snacks. Do not allow the child to snack all day. Meals should have a time limit of 20-30 minutes without distractions such as TV. Solids should be served first followed by liquids so the child does not fill up on liquids. Provide only positive reinforcement, not negative. The number of caregivers involved in feeding should be limited and the expectations should be similar between caregivers.

Characteristics of a breastfed infant

A breastfed infant with growth failure will often be lethargic, sleepy, fussy and cry frequently. Feeding sessions may be very short and the infant may often fall asleep at the breast. Alternately, feeding sessions can be very long but the infant may not be nursing more than 8 times per day. The infant may have very few wet diapers and other signs of dehydration may be present. Maternal factors can sometime be associated with growth failure. This can include inadequate milk production and ineffective milk ejection reflex. Poor milk production can be related to a variety of factors including poor maternal diet, maternal illness, mastitis, fatigue and stress. Psychological factors can also affect milk supply such as if a women feels pressured to breastfeed by family or friends or a negative view of breastfeeding by her partner. Hormonal imbalance and prior breast surgery can play a role. Feeding difficulties such as poor latch, incorrect positioning or infrequent nursing sessions may impair success of breastfeeding. The assistance of a certified lactation consultant is recommended.

Hyperlipidemia

Adolescents and children older than 2 with a total cholesterol greater than 200 or an elevated LDL cholesterol greater than 110 mg/dl should begin the American Heart Association Step I diet for 3 months. The overall goals for Step 1 diet is less than 30% of total calories as fat, less than 10% of total calories as saturated fat, up to 10% of total calories as polyunsaturated fat with the remainder as monounsaturated fat. Trans fats should be avoided. Less than 300 mg of dietary cholesterol is recommended. Calories should be calculated to achieve or maintain an appropriate body weight and to continue to grow and develop normally. If after 3 months, lipid levels do not improve, the Step II diet should be implemented. This diet reduces saturated fat to less than 7% of total calories and restricts cholesterol to less than 200 mg per day. If after 6-12 months lipid levels are still not optimal, medication may need to be considered in children over 10.

National Cholesterol Education Program

The National Cholesterol Education Program (NCEP) recommends that certain children be screened for hyperlipidemia. These include any child over the age of 2 whose parents or grandparents had developed cardiac disease prior to age 55. It also includes children over the age of 2 who have one parent with a total cholesterol greater than 240 mg/dl. Once the child is screened, if total cholesterol is less than 170 mg/dl, basic education on risk reduction should be completed and total cholesterol rechecked in 5 years. If the child's cholesterol is greater than 200 mg/dl, a full lipoprotein analysis should be completed. Education on a Step 1 diet and risk reduction should be completed. If the child's total cholesterol is 170-199 mg/dl, the value should be rechecked then the two results averaged together.

Childhood obesity

Childhood obesity is becoming an epidemic. It is the most common pediatric nutritional issue in the United States. Up to 30% of children and adolescents may be affected. According to the most recent NHANES IV data from 1999-2002, there has been a 3.2% increase in obesity for children ages 2-5, a 4% increase for children ages 6-11, and a 5% increase for children ages 12-19 since the last NHANES III data in 1988-1994. According to NHANES IV, 16% of children ages 6-19 or 9 million children are overweight meaning their body mass index for age is greater than the 95%ile. An additional 15% were at risk for becoming overweight meaning their body mass index for age was between 85-94%ile. The NHANES data also shows that ethnic minorities such as African-American and Mexican-American children have a much higher rate of obesity (20 and 23%) than non-Hispanic white children (14%). Overweight and obese children and adolescents are very likely to remain overweight or obese as adults (70-80% chance).

Complications

Children or adolescents who are overweight or obese are at a much higher risk for developing hypercholesterolemia and hypertension. According to the Bogalusa Heart Study, overall cardiac risk increases from 27% in a non-overweight child to 61% for a child who is overweight. Obese children are also more likely to develop pulmonary complications such as asthma, sleep apnea, hypoventilation syndrome or exercise intolerance. In terms of the musculoskeletal system, a common injury with overweight teens is called slipped capital femoral epiphysis which is when the top of the femur slips out of place before the plates in the hip fuse. Osteoarthritis is also a possibility. There are a variety of mental health issues that can occur when a child is overweight or obese. These can include depression, low self-esteem, poor self-image and peer rejection.

The development of metabolic syndrome is increasing significantly in obese children and adolescents. The characteristics of metabolic syndrome include abdominal obesity, hypertension, hyperlipidemia, and glucose intolerance. Children are considered to have metabolic syndrome if they meet 3 of the following: body mass index above the 97% for age, triglycerides greater than 95%, HDL less than 5% for age, blood pressure greater than the 95% and impaired glucose tolerance. Many of the children with metabolic syndrome will most likely develop type 2 diabetes quickly. The American Diabetes Association has reported that of the new cases of diabetes in children, 45% are type 2. This is almost entirely the result of childhood obesity. Polycystic Ovary Syndrome (PCOS) is another endocrine disorder that often times presents in overweight girls starting at puberty. PCOS can lead to infertility, acne, insulin resistance, and male pattern hair growth.

Nutrition assessment

The nutrition assessment of an obese child should encompass many components.

- Medical history- the presence of medical complications will significantly impact treatment. These complications may include but are not limited to hypertension, diabetes or insulin resistance, pulmonary issues, elevated lipids, and polycystic ovary disease.

- Physical assessment- height and weight should be measured and plotted on NCHS growth charts. Body Mass Index (BMI) should be calculated with a BMI 85-94% for age at risk for becoming overweight and above the 95% for age as overweight. Children who increase 3-4 units of BMI per year are also at risk.

- Nutrition history- a full diet history should be conducted including interviewing the child and parents/caregivers, food frequency and food records. The use of sweetened beverages, eating out and use of take out foods and how food is prepared at home should be closely noted.

- Activity level- assessment of the child's exercise habits and barriers to exercising or increasing physical activity should be noted. The amount of sedentary activity such as computer, television or video game use should also be assessed.

- Support system- an overall assessment of how ready the child and parents are to make the appropriate changes necessary for successful weight management. If a child is not ready, failure can significantly impact the child's self-esteem, may indirectly cause additional weight gain and may jeopardize future attempts. If the family is not ready, the child may not be successful, as he/she may not have alternative supports.

- Environment- this plays a role pivotal role in the lifestyle choices made by the child. Factors to consider are food availability, who cares for the child at various times throughout the day, income levels, and family schedules.

- Psychosocial- these factors can significantly affect the child's ability to change. Factors can include depression, peer rejection/lack of social network, or family issues.

Pediatric obesity

Body mass index (BMI) is a tool for assessing weight status. For children, a BMI between 85-94% indicates the child is at risk for overweight, and a BMI greater than 95% is considered overweight. A measurement of greater than the 95% for age and sex for triceps skinfold is indicative of obesity. A relative weight of 120-140% above ideal body weight is considered mildly obese, 150-199% of ideal body weight is considered moderately obese and greater than 200% is considered severely obese. In terms of growth chart data, using the NCHS growth charts, if a child's weight crosses 2 major percentiles, obesity is probable.

Weight goals

For children ages 2-7 in the 85-94% for BMI, weight goals are for weight maintenance whether or not medical complications are present. With weight maintenance, current body weight is stabilized while linear growth increases allowing the height to catch up to the weight. For BMI greater than 95%, the goal is weight maintenance if medical complications are not present and weight loss if medical complications are present. The weight loss should occur at a rate of 1-2 pounds per month with a goal to reduce BMI to less than 85%. This slow, gradual weight loss will allow body fat to decrease without compromising growth or the building of lean body mass. For children ages 7 years and older with BMI 85-94%, the goal is weight maintenance if no medical complications are present, and weight loss if medical complications are present. For BMI greater than 95%, the goal is for weight loss with or without medical complications. Weight loss should also occur at a rate of 1-2 pounds per month with a desired BMI of less than 85%.

Dietary guidelines

The United States Department of Agriculture began issuing nutrition guidelines in 1894, and in 1943 the department began promoting the Basic 7 food groups. In 1956, Basic 7 was replaced with the Basic Four food groups. These were fruits and vegetables, cereals and breads, milk, and meat. Basic Four lasted until 1992, when it was replaced with the Food Pyramid, which divided food into six groups: 1) Bread, cereal, rice, pasta 2) Fruit 3) Vegetables 4) Meat, poultry, fish, dry beans, eggs, nuts 5) Milk, yogurt, cheese 6) Fats, oils, sweets. The Food Pyramid also provided recommendations for the number of daily servings from each group.

The USDA's Food Pyramid was heavily criticized for being vague and confusing, and in 2011 it was replaced with MyPlate. MyPlate is much easier to understand, as it consists of a picture of a dinner plate divided into four sections, visually illustrating how our daily diet should be distributed among the various food groups. Vegetables and grains each take up 30% of the plate, while fruits and proteins each constitute 20% of the plate. There is also a representation of a cup, marked Dairy, alongside the plate. The idea behind MyPlate is that it's much easier for people to grasp the idea that half of a meal should consist of fruits and vegetables than it is for them to understand serving sizes for all the different kinds of foods they eat on a regular basis.

Obesity treatment

In the age group of 1-5 years, the parents must be the focus of education and behavior modification. Parents are the main influence on what a child eats at this stage and parents still have the most control of eating patterns. For children 5-8 years old, the parents remain the main focus but the children need to begin to learn how to make appropriate food choices for situations where the parent is not present. For children 8-12 years old, the children can begin to take a bigger role for their own weight management. They can begin to practice self-monitoring and goal setting. Children in this age group can better understand the impact of exercise, begin to respond to peer criticism and develop a desire to look better on their own. Children 13 and older should be able to be self-motivated and able to manage their own food choices with some parental support.

Interventions

Parental involvement/behavior modification- this is extremely important in successful pediatric weight management. Both the child and the parents need to be ready to make the appropriate lifestyle changes. The key aspects of this approach is effective nutrition education, education on lifestyle and the risk for developing chronic diseases, and modifying the child's environment at home and school (i.e. removing inappropriate food items, learning healthy cooking techniques, etc.) Other aspects include self-monitoring, parental modeling of appropriate behavior and the use of contracts to promote motivation. The whole family should be committed to weight management for the long term. Physical activity is also an approach to weight management that involves trying to add more physical activity into daily life such as using stairs instead of an elevator, walking more instead of driving). It also tries to encourage less sedentary activities such as television and computer use. One key factor to this approach is parental modeling of increasing physical activity as well as the child. The goal is a minimum of 30 minutes per day three times per week.

Pharmacotherapy and gastric bypass

Pharmacotherapy is an approach that combines intensive behavior modification with appetite suppressing medications. There are currently no drugs approved as safe for use in the pediatric population. Gastric bypass is a surgical procedure that is reserved for morbidly obese adolescents who have been unsuccessful at other concerted efforts at weight loss with diet and behavior modification. This is not a commonly used treatment option at this time but is increasingly becoming an option. This surgery should only be done by a specially trained surgeon and preferably at a center with appropriately trained support staff that has experience in working with adolescents. These children should receive extensive screening by the psychologist, social worker, and RD prior to surgery. Long-term follow-up is extremely important and integral to success. Complications of gastric bypass in teens can include deficiencies of iron, folate, and vitamin D. Malnutrition, chronic diarrhea and vomiting, and cholelithiasis can also develop.

Cardiac lesions

Cardiac lesions are classified into two different types: cyanotic and acyanotic. Children with cyanotic lesion such as Tetralogy of Fallot, Transposition of Great Arteries, pulmonary atresia, and hypoplastic left heart syndrome will typically demonstrate a reduction in both height and weight. If pulmonary hypertension is also present, these children are more likely to be malnourished and have failure to thrive. Acyanotic lesions be due to left to right shunting such as patent ductus arteriosus, ventricular septal defect, atrial septal defect, or AV canal defect. Children with these types of lesions will have difficulty gaining weight. Other acyanotic lesions due to left heart abnormalities include aortic regurgitation, aortic stenosis, and coarctation of the aorta. Children with these types of lesions will typically have more difficulty with linear growth than with weight gain. The timing of the operative repair will also significantly impact the child's nutritional status. Conditions such as hypoplastic left heart syndrome requiring staged repairs will continue to be at risk for compromised growth or failure to thrive between surgeries.

Congenital heart disease

Growth failure

The reasons for growth failure in children with Congenital heart disease (CHD) are multifactorial and include:

- Type of cardiac lesion- cyanotic versus acyanotic
- Increased energy demands due to an increase in basal metabolic rate, increase in total energy output due to increased work of breathing, increased cardiac output. Infection can also increase energy requirements as well as prematurity.
- Decrease in energy intake as a result of poor appetite related to illness, early satiety, too tired to eat adequately related to the heart defect. This can also be due to gastroesophageal reflux or difficulty swallowing.
- Increases in nutrient losses due to malabsorption, the u se of hyperosmolar formulas, poor blood perfusion to the gut, delayed gastric emptying, hepatomegaly related to CHD which in turn decreases gastric capacity. The use of diuretics may increase renal losses of certain electrolytes and minerals.

- The presence of genetic conditions such as Trisomy 21 or other syndrome will affect growth and nutritional status.

Assessment

A comprehensive nutritional assessment of an infant with CHD is essential. The following components should be included:

- Medical history- a detailed history is required that includes the type of cardiac lesion and how old the child was at diagnosis. A complete medication list is essential to assess for any drug nutrient interaction or nutrient losses.
- Physical exam- anthropometric data should be assessed and plotted on NCHS growth chart, which should also include past growth data and growth history. The infant's fluid status should be assessed looking for the presence of edema and urine output should be evaluated. Recent weight trends and observing for signs of congestive heart failure such as diaphoresis, tachypnea and tachycardia should be noted. If fluid overloaded, a dry weight is necessary for calculating medication doses and fluid allotment.
- Laboratory data- the following biochemical indices should be evaluated: serum electrolytes, blood urea nitrogen, creatinine, calcium, phosphorus, magnesium and albumin; urine sodium, potassium, calcium, specific gravity, hemoglobin, hematocrit, iron studies and liver function tests.

Nutritional assessment

Feeding and diet history of the infant with CHD is extremely important. This should also include how well the child feeds, how long the feeding session takes, and the ability to adequately breathe while feeding. This would also include observing breathing patterns, observing the suck-swallow- breathe reflex, monitoring oxygen saturation and respiratory rate during feeding if able, and noting any coughing or vomiting while feeding. The type of formula and the caloric density needs to be obtained as well as the recipe, exact measurements and an assessment of the parent/caregiver's ability to properly make the formula. The review of GI symptoms should include an assessment of formula tolerance, signs of malabsorption such as diarrhea, presence of early satiety and appetite level. Signs of delayed gastric emptying, GE reflux or aspiration should be noted. Additional work up by a pediatric GI specialist may be warranted based on the severity of symptoms and growth.

Tube feeding

Tube feeding is an important option to provide total or partial nutrition to a child with CHD. Indications for tube feeding may include failure to thrive, inability to consume adequate nutrition by mouth because of appetite limitations or limited endurance. Options for initiating tube feedings can include continuous, bolus or nocturnal tube feedings. Bolus feedings are more physiologic but continuous may be better tolerated in this population because of the risk for aspiration and GI issues such as delayed gastric emptying. Nocturnal tube feedings would allow a child to eat during the day and receive supplemental tube feedings at night at the desired calorie level. Contraindications to tube feedings would include active GI bleeding, bowel obstruction, low cardiac output, or hemodynamic instability. Gut perfusion may be affected.

Transition from parenteral to enteral nutrition

Parenteral nutrition (PN) is often required for children with CHD who are acutely ill in the hospital. PN is indicated until enteral nutrition (EN) is able to advance towards goal. Because decreased gut perfusion may be an issue, transition from PN to EN should occur slowly. Trophic feedings are useful in infants with GI issues due to CHD. As EN increases, the amount of PN can be inversely decreased to prevent volume overload. Once the infant reaches full volume of EN, PN can be discontinued. The caloric density of the formula or breast milk can be gradually increased by 1-2 kcal/ounce per day. If using infant formula, it can be concentrated to provide the same ratio of protein, fat and carbohydrate, or modular products can be added. Caloric density of up to 30 kcal/ounce is often required. Caution should be taken with medications as many are hyperosmolar and may cause GI distress.

Calorie and protein requirements

The presence of malnutrition is high in infants and children with CHD. The best gauge for assessing the adequacy of calorie intake is to estimate needs using a predictive equation then follow growth parameters. Calorie requirements will vary but infants with CHD typically require 130-155 kcal/kg. Children may need 20-30% above the RDA. After cardiac repair, calorie requirements will be less but may remain 10-15 kcal/kg above the RDA. The overall goal is for normal growth and development. Protein requirements can generally be met with the RDA for age. Micronutrient intake should be carefully calculated to ensure that there is no deficiency that may affect growth. Supplements should be given as needed.

Developmental disability

Developmental disability is defines as any congenital or acquired condition that affects intellectual or cognitive ability, growth and development. This is often referred to as children with special health care needs. Children with developmental disabilities often have oral motor problems. This can include a weak suck, impaired swallow ability, tongue thrusting, excessive drool, choking, and hyperactive gag. Because of the developmental disability, these children often lag behind children of normal abilities in the development of certain feeding skills. Factors to consider when assessing feeding skills include the age of the child versus the developmental age, what feeding techniques have worked in the past, what is the best position to feed the child in, and evaluation of dental health. Sensory responses such as visual or auditory cues or stimuli, the smell or taste of certain foods, and temperature sensitivity should be evaluated. A team approach is best when performing feeding assessments for children with special health care needs. The team should include an RD, occupational therapist, physical therapist, speech pathologist, psychologist or social worker and physician.

Assessment of calorie requirements

Calorie requirements for children with developmental disabilities can vary greatly. Calorie requirements are often lower than children with normal abilities because the growth rate is lower, activity levels are often lower, and basal metabolic rate may be lower. This may apply to children with Down syndrome, Prader Willi, and spina bifida. Other children may have higher than normal calorie requirements because of increased activity such as spasticity, children with seizures or cerebral palsy. A comprehensive weight and growth history, diet and feeding history should be completed. The RDA is often a starting point, however, the use of height age may be a better way to assess calorie requirements than actual age. Alternately, calculating energy requirements based on calories per centimeter may provide greater accuracy. Overall, calorie intake and growth patterns should be reviewed frequently and readjusted as needed to help prevent over or under nutrition.

Down syndrome

Children with Down syndrome (DS) or Trisomy 21 are often born with medical issues such as heart defects or problems with their GI tract. Many of these issues can now be detected prenatally. During the first year of life, children with DS are at risk for poor weight gain. This is mainly due to hypotonia, poor feeding skills or other medical issues that may be present. As the child gets older, growth concerns will shift to risk for obesity. This is related to decreased activity levels, lower basal metabolic requirements and low muscle tone. Growth should be monitored closely for weight for age, length or height for age, head circumference for children younger than 3, weight for length or body mass index. Height is compromised. Weight for height and/or body mass index is usually elevated unless closely monitored with appropriate intervention. Calorie requirements are based on height per centimeter rather than weight. Children with DS can also have issues with constipation due to low muscle tone, decreased activity and possible poor fiber and/or fluid intake.

Anthropometric measurements

Anthropometric data is extremely important in the nutritional assessment of children with developmental delay. These measurements may be difficult to obtain, however, due to impaired gross motor skills or inability to stand on own. There are several types of scales available for obtaining weight including chair, bucket or bed scales. For assessing height, arm span, sitting height or knee to ankle height may be used. There are growth charts available for a variety of developmental delays such as Down syndrome or cerebral palsy, however, the use of CDC growth charts is recommended. Many of the specialty growth charts were developed using a small sample size. Careful interpretation of growth curves is needed. Finally, because height tends to be lower than average, close monitoring of weight for height or body mass index is required. Many children with developmental delay have decreased muscle mass, which will impact interpretation of the body mass index. Mid arm muscle circumference and triceps skin fold are also a useful tool for assessment.

Nutrition care plan

After the nutritional issues have been determined, the next step is implementation. Factors to consider include:

- Interest and motivation level of the family or caregiver. Also, the education level and the family's ability to understand and implement the plan needs to be taken into account
- Prioritizing points in the nutrition plan is important. Often times, families are only able to address one issue at a time or only give 1-2 issues to work on initially to prevent families from becoming overwhelmed.
- Available community resources to assist with the cost should be explored. Early Intervention programs are available in all states and include nutrition services. Schools need to accommodate diet modifications if prescribed by a physician because of the Individuals with Disabilities Act. Also, other assistance such as WIC or food stamps may be a possible resource.

Cystic Fibrosis

Nutrition therapy

Nutrition goals for children with Cystic Fibrosis (CF) include improved survival, normal growth and development and to prevent and treat malnutrition. Children with CF should follow a diet that is high in calories and protein. Many patients with CF will be able to grow normally with a calorie level close to the RDA. Some patients, however, will require 20-50% more. Protein should be calculated are 1.5-2 times the RDA with severe disease. In the past, a fat restriction was recommended but should now be provided at 35-45% if total calories. Increasing the fat content of the diet also helps with increasing the calorie content. Children with CF need to take additional amounts of the fat-soluble vitamins A, D, E, and K. This is given as a multivitamin supplement such as ADEK or SourceCF softgel. Children should consume the DRI's for other vitamins and minerals. Calcium is particularly important as children with CF are at risk for decreased bone density. Additional sodium is sometimes required during hot weather, increased activity, with fever or diarrhea

Clinical manifestations

There are many clinical manifestations of CF and these can vary from one child to another. Approximately 85% of children with CF have pancreatic involvement that can lead to gastrointestinal complications. The nutritional effects of pancreatic involvement are malabsorption of fat, fat-soluble vitamins and essential fatty acids, and protein.

Gastrointestinal complications can include failure to thrive, steatorrhea, foul smelling stools, anorexia, bile salt and bile acid deficiency which can also contribute to fat soluble vitamin deficiency. Pulmonary manifestations include chronic cough, chronic pulmonary infections, difficulty breathing, bronchospasms and chronic sinusitis. The nutritional effects of pulmonary involvement includes increasing caloric requirements related to increased work of breathing and increased coughing, and fatigue which can lead to decreased intake. Chronic pulmonary infections can also increase caloric needs. Chronic coughing can lead to a cough-emesis cycle that can affect intake.

Growth patterns

A chronic calorie deficit may be present due to effects of the disease and an increase in resting energy expenditure. Catch up growth is often required. The majority of CF patients are smaller in stature and weigh less than other children their age. Growth failure is correlated with the severity of pulmonary complications. One study done in 1993 based on the CF Foundation national patient registry found that the median height for age and weight for age was the 20th percentile on NCHS growth charts. The 2002 CF Foundation patient registry details 17% of patients with CF had weights less than 5th percentile and almost 16% has heights less than the 5th percentile.

Nutritional failure

Children with CF are considered to have nutritional failure of length or height is less than 5th percentile, percentage of ideal body weight is less than 90% of predicted, weight for length in children ages 0-2 years is less than 10th percentile and body mass index for children ages 2-20 is less than 10th percentile for age. Many studies have documented the use of nutritional status as a significant prognostic indicator. For example, children at age 3 with good growth parameters had better lung function at age 6. Also, patients with CF whose weight for height was 90% of predicted had lower pulmonary function tests than those with normal weights. Being underweight is a negative prognostic indicator. Height has also been found to be a prognostic indicator for survival.

Anthropometric information

Growth parameters are extremely important components of a nutritional assessment of a child with CF. For children less than 3 years of age, a weight for age, length for age, weight for height and head circumference should be measured and plotted on a NCHS growth chart. For children older than 2 y ears, height for age if able to stand, and weight for age should be obtained and plotted. Body mass index for age should be calculated and plotted as well. The RD should also calculate the child's weight as a percentage of ideal weight for height. This can be determined by finding the height age or the age where the height is at the 50% then extrapolating the weight from the growth chart. At least yearly, mid arm muscle circumference and triceps skin folds should be measured and compared to data for age and gender. One other measurement that can be obtained is the mid-parental height to see if the child with CF is achieving full height potential.

Vitamin assays and iron studies

Laboratory data is an important component of the nutritional assessment of a child with CF. The CF foundation has developed guidelines for monitoring. Vitamins A, D, E and K should be checked at diagnosis then yearly. Vitamin A should not be checked during acute illness as it is a negative acute phase reactant and may be falsely low because of this. Vitamin A can be checked as retinol, Vitamin D as 25-OH vitamin D and vitamin E as alpha-tocopherol. The prothrombin time can be monitored as a marker for vitamin K status especially for those children on long-term antibiotics that may be at risk for vitamin K deficiency due to changes in gut flora. Iron status should be checked at diagnosis then every year using hemoglobin and hematocrit. If anemia is present, additional iron studies should be obtained including serum iron, iron binding capacity, ferritin, and reticulocyte count.

Biochemical data

Other lab data to be monitored include protein status. This should be assessed at diagnosis then annually. Protein status should be monitored more closely if the child has malnutrition or growth failure. Albumin is generally the marker that is checked. Sodium can be checked as needed but especially during extreme heat or dehydration. Breast fed infants should have sodium monitored. Zinc is difficult to assess biochemically but can be considered if the child is experiencing growth failure. Essential fatty acid deficiency can be checked in infants or children with growth failure. This can be measured by checking the triene to tetraene ration that will be decreased with deficiency. Blood glucose levels should be monitored annually at the least to screen for CF related diabetes (CFRD).

Clinical assessment

The physician and/or nurse should complete the general review of systems although the RD can also do a visual assessment. The clinical information important to the RD's assessment includes:

- Information from the review of systems including pulmonary status including pulmonary function tests, presence of infection, GE reflux.
- General activity and energy level and if CF has been affecting daily life such as missing school or work.
- Stool pattern, which would include frequency, consistency, characteristics such as color, oily, foul smelling, abdominal cramping.
- Enzyme therapy that would include the type, dose, brand, when they are taken, and how they are taken in relation to meals. The units of lipase per kilogram body weight per meal should be calculated.
- The use of other medications such as diuretics, steroids, antibiotics, antacids, etc
- The use of alternative medicine
- Vitamin and mineral supplementation including doses and compliance
- Drug nutrient interactions

Diet history

A thorough diet history should be completed. There are several methods that can be used to assess diet history. This includes 3-5 day food records, 24 hour recall and food frequency questionnaire. The use of nutritional supplements should be assessed and documented. The RD should calculate the nutritional adequacy of the diet especially for calories, protein, calcium, iron, and other vitamins and minerals. The percentage of fat should be calculated. Information on appetite, meal pattern, and schedule and any behavioral issues should be assessed. For children who receive tube feedings, a thorough assessment should be completed including product used, volume taken per day, tolerance, type of feeding tube and compliance. Vitamin and mineral supplement use and compliance should be assessed as well as the use of any alternative medicine such as herbs.

Cystic Fibrosis Related Diabetes

As children with CF get older, the risk for developing Cystic Fibrosis Related Diabetes

(CFRD) increases. CFRD is often the cause for unexplained weight loss and lack of energy in adolescents or young adults with CF. It is believed to be caused by a decreased ability of the pancreas to produce sufficient insulin as a result of damage to the islet cells. The islet cells are the cells in the pancreas that produce insulin and these get damaged because of abnormal secretions and scarring in the pancreas. Insulin resistance is also present. CFRD is different than type 1 or 2 diabetes. Annual screening is recommended. A random blood glucose level greater than 126 mg/dl indicates the need for additional testing.

Blood glucose level

Next, a fasting blood glucose should be checked. If this is also greater than 126 mg/dl and a random blood glucose is greater than 200 mg/dl, CFRD can be diagnosed. An oral glucose tolerance test should be done for any patient with signs of diabetes such as polydipsia or polyuria if fasting blood glucose is normal. The elevated energy needs for CF needs to be prioritized over the CF related diabetes. Nutrition intervention should include an appropriate calorie level, timing of meals and snacks in relation to insulin regimen, and enzyme supplementation. The insulin requirements need to be individually tailored to meet the needs for CF. Diagnosing CFRD early is the goal to prevent weight loss in a population that cannot afford to lose any weight.

Osteopenia

Osteopenia and osteoporosis is a clinical concern for patients with CF. Children with CF may have one or more of the following risk factors in their medical history: failure to thrive, low weight for height (body mass index less than 25% or weight for length less than 25%), delayed puberty which impacts skeletal and sexual maturation, malabsorption of key nutrients for bone health or the use of steroids for lung disease for more than 3 months in the past year. Poor intake of calcium or vitamin D as well as low serum 25-OH vitamin D levels also increases the risk. Low vitamin K levels will also impact bone health. Children over the age of 8 and who have one or more risk factors should have a bone mass assessment done by DEXA scan. Additionally, children should have yearly monitoring of serum calcium, phosphorus, parathyroid hormone and 25-OH vitamin D levels.

Breastfeeding

An infant with CF is at risk for developing malnutrition due to the need for rapid growth, brain development and increased energy levels. Essential fatty acid deficiency is common and should always be assessed with infant experiencing growth failure. Breast milk is the preferred food for infants during the first year. Infants with CF can achieve normal growth and development with the proper use of pancreatic enzymes. Close monitoring of protein status is necessary as breast milk is lower in protein than infant formula although it is typically better absorbed. If the infant requires additional calories, supplementing breastfeeding with calorically dense breast milk or infant formula may be an option. Hyponatremic alkalosis is also a concern as the sodium content is lower in breast milk than infant formula. Sodium supplementation in the form of NaCl is generally required for breast fed infants.

Formula feeding

If breast milk is not available, infant formula is the appropriate substitution. Cow's milk based formulas can be used if appropriate pancreatic enzyme replacement is provided. The infant should be monitored closely for appropriate growth and evidence of fat malabsorption that would include frequent, loose stools that are oily. If an infant has required a bowel resection due to meconium ileus that is often seen in newborns with CF, a formula with hydrolyzed protein and medium chain triglycerides such as Pregestimil or Alimentum should be used. The caloric density of the formula will typically need to be increased for 24-30 kcal/ounce depending upon calorie requirements and growth. This can be done by concentration and/or the addition of modular products.

Introduction of solid food

Solid food can be introduced when the infant is developmentally ready, usually around 4-6 months of age. Introducing infant cereal first is recommended followed by strained fruits, vegetables and meats. New foods should be added one at a time while observing for adverse reactions. Calories can be increased in strained foods if needed by adding fat or carbohydrate modulars. Cereal can be mixed with breast milk or infant formula to maximize nutrient content. Pancreatic enzyme replacement should be adjusted as needed to allow for maximum fat absorption. Gastroesophageal reflux (GER) is commonly seen in infants with CF. This may cause weight loss or growth failure if severe enough, and it may also exacerbate pulmonary issues. Infants with GER will have reduced feeding volumes, arching of back, vomiting and possible growth failure. Appropriate management should be implemented.

Toddler or preschool age children

Toddlers and preschool age children with CF have the same issues transitioning to table food and developing healthy eating habits as children without CF do. The main difference is the children with CF have the risk of developing malnutrition. A normal slowing of growth occurs during this period and activity levels will increase. Appetite level decreases and providing adequate calories for a child with CF can be a challenge. Regular meals and snacks should be offered and children should not be allowed to graze throughout the day. Prevention of mealtime stress is important as it may lead to behavioral issues or disordered eating. A plan needs to be made for the child to take pancreatic enzyme replacement at school or daycare. If growth is compromised despite providing a high calorie, high protein diet with appropriate pancreatic enzyme replacement, nutritional supplements such as a milk shake made with instant breakfast powder or a commercial product made need to be initiated.

Children ages 6-18 years

Starting at around age 6, children need to begin to take more responsibility for self-care and monitoring. This should include selecting own food choices and learning how to prepare quick, high calorie foods and snacks. Calorie requirements can be 20-50% above the RDA. Some children in this age group require supplemental tube feedings to meet calorie requirements for growth. Good nutrition promotes better weight status and lung function, which are closely related. Children with CF should be monitored every 3 months for adequate diet, nutritional status and growth. Attaining normal bone mass is essential to long-term bone health. Puberty can be delayed by poor growth or poor nutrition. Any weight loss in teenagers should be evaluated. Pulmonary status should be closely monitored. Screening for CF related diabetes (CFRD) should continue. Adolescents should also be monitored for depression and disordered eating. Compliance with vitamins and pancreatic enzyme replacement should be followed.

Pancreatic enzyme replacement therapy

Pancreatic enzymes contain amylase for carbohydrate digestion and absorption, lipase for fat, and proteases for protein. They come as enteric-coated microspheres, microtablets or powder. Applesauce is often used to mix with the enzymes in infants and young children because an acidic pH is required in the stomach to activate the enzymes. Enzymes should be dosed according to the child's weight, composition of diet and portion sizes. Dosage can be based on lipase units per kilogram of body weight or on grams of long chain fat. A typical starting dose for an infant is 2000 units of lipase per 4 ounces of formula or one breastfeeding session. For children ages 1-4, the dose may start at 1000 units per meal. For children older than 4 years, the dose may start at 500 units per kg per meal. Doses for snacks are usually half of the meal dose. Enzymes should be taken just before meals and snacks. Careful monitoring of growth and GI symptoms will help to ensure the correct dose is provided.

Pancreatic enzyme replacement and tube feedings

Many children with CF require gastrostomy tubes for supplemental nutrition. Often times the child is receiving a continuous infusion that creates problems for enzyme dosing as enzymes are meant to be given at individual meals. Selection of formula can vary from polymeric with intact protein to formulas with varying caloric concentrations to partially hydrolyzed formulas. The partially hydrolyzed formulas contain more MCT oil to help with fat absorption and may also reduce the amount of enzyme replacement needed. Doses are based on the amount of long chain fats in the formula. 1000- 2000 units of lipase per gram of long chain fat is a safe starting dose. The enzymes can be taken orally and care must be taken when administering via the feeding tube as it may clog or cause other problems. Doses for continuous tube feedings can be divided into 2/3 before the feeding and 1/3 at the end. Bolus feedings are easier to manage as the enzymes can be given followed by the bolus.

Vitamin supplementation

Vitamin and mineral supplements are required by all children with CF and pancreatic insufficiency. If liver disease is also present, the risk for fat-soluble vitamin deficiency is even greater. Specific vitamin supplements designed for use in patients with CF are available. The fat-soluble vitamins are provided in the water-soluble form to assist with absorption. These vitamins include Vitamin A, D, E, and K along with B vitamins. Vitamin A is important for sight, skin integrity and immune function. Requirements are for age 0-1= 1500 units, age 1-3= 5000 units, age 4-8= 5000-10,000 units and for ages 8 and older= 10,000 units. Vitamin D is important to help prevent osteopenia, osteoporosis, and bone fractures. The requirements are for age 0-1= 400 units and 400-800 units for children older than 1 year.

Vitamin K deficiency is common due to altered gut flora and may cause coagulopathy. Supplementing vitamin K improves prothrombin time. Requirements are 0.3-0.5 mg and 5-10 mg is given to correct deficiency. Vitamin E is needed as an antioxidant, helps to protect cell membranes such as in lungs from oxidative damage, and for immune function. A separate vitamin E supplement is often needed in addition to the multivitamin preparation to meet requirements of age 0-1 year = 40-50 units, 1-3 years = 0-150 units, 4-8 years= 100-200 units and older than 8 years= 200-400 units. Water-soluble vitamins should be provided at 2 times the DRI and can be met with a combination of diet and the use of multivitamin product for CF patients such as ADEK, Vitamax or Source CF softgels. Zinc is often included in the multivitamin preparation.

Growth failure

Growth failure is commonly referred to as failure to thrive and is poor growth occurring during the first 3 years of life. A universal and exact method for identifying growth failure has not been established. Commonly used criteria for identifying growth failure include: weight for age less than the 3rd or 5th percentile on the NCHS growth charts; weight for length or weight for height less than the 3rd or 5th percentile; a decrease in growth rate over 2 major percentiles for 3-6 months; a decrease of 2 standard deviations on the NCHS growth chart over 3-6 months. It is important to note that a pattern of growth is the best way to assess growth trends. A single plot on a growth chart does not give any information on growth rate or pattern.

Weight for age and linear growth

One point of view regarding weight for age is that an infant's weight percentile at 1-2 months is a better indicator of weight percentile at 12 months than is the birth weight percentile. For the long term, however, weight for age alone cannot be used as the only criteria for growth failure as the child may also have a low length or height for age. In this case, the actual weight for length or weight for height may be appropriate. Children with this scenario may just be genetically small or had issues earlier in life but may not be acutely malnourished now. Linear growth should be evaluated along with genetic growth potential by noting parental height. Premature and small for gestational age infants should be carefully evaluated.

Organic growth failure

Organic growth failure occurs because of a medical condition that interferes with intake, absorption, or utilization of nutrients. Organic growth failure can be the inability to consume enough calories because of a neurological impairment or problems with sucking, swallowing or chewing. It can be due to the inability of the body to use the nutrients because of vomiting, gastroesophageal reflux, or malabsorption from inflammatory bowel disease, celiac disease, Cystic Fibrosis, or short gut syndrome. It can also be caused by increased energy requirements in conditions such as congenital heart disease, bronchopulmonary dysplasia or persistent fevers. One other possibility can be conditions where growth potential is altered such as prematurity or intrauterine growth restriction, congenital anomalies, chromosomal or genetic disorders, in-born errors of metabolism, or endocrine disorders such as hypothyroidism or growth hormone deficiency.

Non-organic growth failure

Non-organic growth failure may be related to social or behavioral issues leading to poor intake. This can be due to the family or caregiver's inability to provide adequate nutrition due to a poor financial situation. Psychosocial issues such as neglect or abuse, a mom who is overwhelmed, drug or alcohol abuse preventing the parent or caregiver from caring appropriately for the child. Increased stress in the home due to chronic illness, marital problems or a history of loss or death can contribute. Non-organic growth failure can also be attributed to improper formula preparation, excessive juice intake, inappropriate feeding practices or atypical health or nutrition practices or beliefs that may impact growth such as fear of the child getting fat or belief that breast milk will sustain nutritional status indefinitely. It can also be caused by a delayed introduction to solids, coercive feeding practices or stressful meal times, or increased amounts of distractions during meals or feeding. Inadequate breast milk production can also be a reason.

GI disorders

Barium swallow- a test that visualizes the upper GI tract and small bowel looking for hiatal hernia, varices or dysmotility disorders.

Esophageal pH monitoring- also called a pH probe where a pH sensor is inserted through the esophagus for 24 hours to monitor for gastroesophageal reflux.

EGD- esophagogastroduodenoscopy, which is a tube that is threaded through the esophagus to the duodenum that visualizes the lining and takes biopsies along the way. This test looks for inflammation such as gastritis, esophagitis or peptic ulcer disease.

Upper GI with small bowel follow through- us a barium study that visualizes the upper GI tract through the small bowel looking for inflammation, strictures, structural lesion.

Barium enema- is a test that visualizes the lower GI tract including the colon and rectum and looks for polyps, colitis, diverticulitis, ulcerative colitis, Hirschsprung's, intestinal obstruction, intussusception.

D-xylose- is a test to check of the presence of malabsorption by giving oral D-xylose and checking for the presence of D-xylose in the blood at high levels (low amounts is abnormal).

Qualitative fecal fat- a 2 day collection of stool ideally using a 100 gram fat test diet. This monitors for fat malabsorption, pancreatic insufficiency, celiac disease.

Abdominal ultrasound- uses sound waves to look at organs and structures in the upper GI tract including the abdomen, liver, and pancreas. This can detect gallstones, biliary tract abnormalities, and tumors.

Colonoscopy- insertion of a fiberoptic tube from the anus to the colon. This visualizes the lining and takes biopsies looking for colitis, polyps, ischemic colitis

Laboratory tests

Serum bilirubin- a blood test that measures the excretory function of the liver and can help diagnose hepatitis, disorders of the biliary tract, cholestasis

Ammonia level- blood test that measures how well the liver is able to breakdown protein for excretion. Serum levels will rise if the liver cannot break down ammonia to urea. This test helps to diagnose hepatic encephalopathy, liver failure, and certain inborn errors of metabolism.

Prothrombin time (PTT)- a blood test the measures the synthetic function of the liver, PTT is dependent on vitamin K and other clotting factors. An elevated PTT can help to determine if hepatic protein synthesis is reduced if the patient is not on antibiotics.

Aminotransferase levels- these include aspartate aminotransferase (AST or SGOT), alanine aminotransferase (ALT or SGPT). This test can help to diagnose hepatitis.

Serum amylase or lipase- these blood tests help to check pancreatic function and can help diagnose inflammation or obstruction, pancreatitis

Crohn's disease and Ulcerative Colitis

Crohn's disease and Ulcerative Colitis (UC) are both types of inflammatory bowel disease (IBD). These two diseases have similar symptoms including GI bleeding, diarrhea, abdominal pain, weight loss and anemia. Crohn's disease can occur in any part of the GI tract while UC occurs only in the colon with minimal involvement of the terminal ileum. Crohn's disease can occur in segments leaving parts of the GI tract unaffected. The terminal ileum is the location most frequently affected in Crohn's disease. UC can be cured with a total colectomy whereas there is no surgical cure available for Crohn's disease, however, remission may be induced with a partial resection of the diseased area. Up to 30% of children with IBD will have growth failure and children with Crohn's are more likely to have linear stunting that does not catch up.

Inflammatory bowel disease

Early nutrition intervention is recommended for children with Inflammatory bowel disease (IBD) to prevent or treat malnutrition and growth failure. Nutrition intervention should be coupled with medical intervention for optimal results. A high calorie, high protein diet that is well balanced is recommended. Any diet restrictions should be determined by the individual child's tolerance. Possible diet modifications include lactose restriction, fiber restriction (especially for children with ulcerative colitis and strictures), and fat restriction if steatorrhea is present. Because weight loss is common in both Crohn's disease and ulcerative colitis, aggressive nutrition therapy to try to reverse any delays on growth should be attempted. This may include the use of enteral nutrition especially for those with Crohn's. Elemental formulas have been tried but are very unpalatable if taken orally even with the addition of flavorings. Nocturnal delivery of elemental formulas by nasogastric or gastrostomy tube has also been used with success. Some children will tolerate a polymeric formula without difficulty. The use of total parenteral nutrition should be used in severe cases that cannot tolerate any enteral nutrition

<u>Vitamin and mineral deficiencies</u>
The presence of malabsorption in IBD may cause deficiencies in vitamins A, C, E, D, K, and folate. Vitamin B12 deficiency is possible especially if the terminal ileum has been removed. Calcium and magnesium deficiency may also be present and can affect bone health long term. Zinc deficiency is possible with the use of corticosteroids, chronic diarrhea and may contribute to growth failure. Anemia is common and should be monitored by checking serum iron, iron binding capacity, and ferritin. A general multivitamin supplement with minerals is recommended for all children with IBD. Zinc should be supplemented at 2

times the DRI if the child is experiencing excessive stool output or has fistula drainage. B12 injections should be given if deficiency is documented. Folate should be supplemented at 1-2 times the DRI as certain medications such as sulfasalazine may interfere with metabolism. A calcium supplement is recommended to meet the DRI especially for children receiving corticosteroids.

Constipation

Constipation in children can involves a decrease in frequency of stool passage to less than 3 per week, passage of very hard stool and can include pain while trying to pass stool even though frequency may be normal. The goal of nutrition therapy is to improve bowel function for softer, more easy to pass stools. For children older than a year, increasing fiber in the diet is the key. The fiber goal should be approximately 0.5 grams/kg per day or another recommendation is the age of the child plus 5 grams. Whole grain breads and cereals, bran, fruits, vegetables, and legumes are all foods that can provide added fiber. For infants experiencing constipation, the use of barley cereal or the addition of prune or pear juice at 2 ml/kg per day may help. Another important key to improving constipation is adequate fluid intake to meet baseline fluid requirements. Increasing activity should also help.

Acute diarrhea

Acute diarrhea is defined as diarrhea occurring for less than 7 days. A diet history should be taken to try to determine if the diarrhea may be related to diet. Consuming too much juice such as apple or pear juice can induce diarrhea because of the high sorbitol content. Occasionally a secondary lactose intolerance due to rotavirus infection may manifest itself temporarily. Nutrition intervention for acute diarrhea involves correcting dehydration. Oral rehydration therapy (ORT) is recommended using a low osmolarity fluid such as Pedialyte or Infalyte. ORT contains potassium, sodium and chloride to help replace excessive losses. Other fluids such as Gatorade, soda, or juice may worsen the problem because of the higher osmolarity. Once food can be reintroduced, the use of complex carbohydrates such as rice, potatoes, bread, cereals, and lean meats, fruits, vegetables and yogurt may be well tolerated. Full strength infant formula or breast milk can also be restarted. The use of the BRAT diet (bananas, rice, applesauce, toast) is often recommended but is of limited nutritional quality.

<u>Chronic diarrhea of infancy</u>

The first step in the nutritional management of chronic diarrhea of infancy is rehydration. The next step involves a slow reintroduction of enteral nutrition or a combination of enteral and parenteral nutrition. Careful monitoring for refeeding syndrome is warranted. Potassium and phosphorus often require supplementation because of this. Daily monitoring of electrolytes including potassium, phosphorus, glucose and magnesium is necessary. Protein, fat and vitamins can be given at levels to meet requirements but carbohydrate needs to be introduced and advanced slowly. For the enterally fed infant, continuous feedings can improve absorption. A lactose free formula may be needed and in certain cases, a semi elemental protein hydrolysate formula such as Alimentum or Pregestimil may be needed. Breast milk if available can also be used in place of formula. If the infant takes solids, infant cereal and other age appropriate foods can be slowly reintroduced. Juice should be avoided because of its high osmotic load. Supplemental zinc can be given at 2-3 times the DRI for oral supplementation.

Short Bowel Syndrome

Short Bowel Syndrome (SBS) is a condition where 40-60% of the small intestine is resected resulting in significant malabsorption of fluid and nutrients. This can occur in the pediatric population as a result of gastroschisis, necrotizing colitis, intestinal atresia, inflammatory bowel disease, radiation enteritis, intestinal pseudo-obstruction, volvulus or vascular infarct. The normal length of the small intestine is in a term infant is approximately 250-300 cm and includes the duodenum, jejunum and ileum. As the child grows, the small intestine will also grow up to an additional 2-3 meters in adulthood. The large intestine is approximately 30-40 cm at birth and will reach a final length of 1.5-2 meters in adulthood. An infant requires approximately 10-30 cm of small intestine with an ileocecal valve but 30-50 cm if the ileocecal valve has been removed.

Clinical outcome

The length of the remaining small intestine will have the greatest impact on clinical outcome. Most digestion occurs in the first 100 cm of the small intestine. If the duodenum is resected, this will affect iron and folate absorption. If the both the duodenum and jejunum are resected, the ileum can assume the functions of both that include the primary absorption site for protein, carbohydrate and fat as well as minerals. Resection of the distal ileum will have the most significant effect pm clinical condition and will most likely result in serious nutritional and medical complications. The distal ileum is the only site for vitamin B12 and bile salt absorption that in turn affects fat and fat-soluble vitamin absorption. It also absorbs a significant amount of fluid. The presence of the ileocecal valve is extremely important as this helps to slow transit time and prevent bacterial overgrowth from occurring.

Nutritional management

Parenteral nutrition is considered the first phase of nutritional management for SBS. PN should be started as soon as possible after resection. Central access should be obtained as quickly as possible to provide appropriate fluid and nutrition support. The initial goal post operatively is fluid and electrolyte replacement. Increased losses of sodium, potassium, and chloride can occur through gastric drainage or ileostomy output. Replacement fluids can be used to replace these losses. Calorie requirements for PN in infants are approximately 90-100 kcal/kg with 3-3.5 grams/kg protein. Older children may require 30-50% above BMR. Additional zinc may be required due to increased stool output. Magnesium deficiency may also occur. The overall goal for PN is to meet appropriate micro and macro nutrient requirements for growth and development without overfeeding and to try to prevent long-term complications of PN such as cholestasis or PN associated liver disease.

The initiation of enteral nutrition is considered the second phase of nutritional management for patients with SBS. Enteral nutrition should begin once GI motility returns and fluid and electrolyte requirements have stabilized. Delays in enteral nutrition are not recommended, as this will delay the start of the adaptive process. The most appropriate formula to use initially remains under debate. For infants, breast milk should be used of available. Not only will the infant receive the many benefits of breast milk including enzymes, growth hormones, nucleotides, etc but it may also stimulate mucosal growth. If breast milk is not available, protein hydrolysate formulas such as Pregestimil or Alimentum can be used for infants or toddlers. Preterm infants with smaller resections may be able to tolerate the reduced lactose content and fat blend of preterm formulas. Toddlers or older children may be able to tolerate a fiber containing polymeric formula such as PediaSure with Fiber.

The third phase of nutritional management is when the bowel has completely adapted and the transition to solid food occurs. Infants can begin solid food at the normally recommended time of 4-6 months. Cereals should be started first and are usually tolerated well. For older children, age appropriate protein containing foods that are lower in fat should be introduced before carbohydrates. Foods with a high osmotic content or simple sugars should be delayed such as juice or sweets. The use of fiber especially soy polysaccharides and pectin can help to lengthen transit time and promote absorption. Fiber also serves as fuel for colonocytes. Once tolerance to initial diet is established, complex carbohydrates can be introduced. The complete transition to oral diet can take weeks to months depending upon tolerance to foods and progress with addressing oral aversion if present. As oral intake improves, supplementation with semi elemental or polymeric formula can begin.

<u>Adaptive changes</u>

After the intestinal resection, the remaining intestine has the ability to take on the role of the resected parts depending upon the area. These changes will begin 12-24 hours following surgery and can continue for over a year. Changes that can occur include increase in bowel length, increase in villi length thus increasing the amount of absorptive area with a gradual increase in the absorptive process. Bowel circumference and bowel wall thickness can also increase. There is also an enhanced hormonal response occurring during adaptation. The most important trigger for the adaptive process to begin is the introduction of enteral nutrition to stimulate mucosal growth. Complex nutrients seem to promote intestinal adaptation better than amino acids or monosaccharides. Glutamine also plays a role. Younger infants have a greater chance for full adaptation because of the chance for additional bowel length as the infant grows.

Tube feeding plan

Children with SBS starting enteral nutrition should have a nasogastric tube placed. Preterm infants should have an orogastric tube, as they are obligate nose breathers. If tube feedings are expected for more than 3 months, a surgically places gastrostomy tube should be placed. The preferred method of tube feeding administration is continuous infusion as it allows for greater nutrient absorption. The tube feeding rate should be gradually advanced to allow for better tolerance. The child should be monitored for the presence of vomiting, increased stool or ostomy output or abdominal distention. Because feeding aversion can occur, a plan for oral stimulation should be in place. Tube feedings can be transitioned to a nocturnal schedule when oral diet begins to help stimulate appetite.

Transitioning from parenteral to enteral nutrition

The biggest factor affecting the transition from PN to EN is time. Transitioning can be a very slow process. Malabsorption is a very common issue. When nutrition is provided parenterally, 100% is absorbed. As enteral nutrition increases, the amount of calories required from enteral nutrition also increases to account for absorption. This also increases caloric requirements approximately 30-50% above basal needs. One recommendation for transitioning is for each 3 cc increase in tube feeding rate, there can be a concurrent 1 cc decrease in PN rate. Lipid infusion can remain constant to provide additional calories. Another option is to wean PN be the same number of calories that the tube feeding has advanced by. The PN rate or the number of hours PN is provided can be reduced. Feeding tolerance needs to be monitored closely. This can be measured by monitoring stool or ostomy output. Once advancement per day is recommended per day of either volume or concentration. If a volume increase is not tolerated, reduce rate then try a change in strength or concentration.

Stool and ostomy output

General guidelines are if the stool output is less than 10 stools per day or less that 10 grams/kg per day, the enteral rate can be increased by 10-20 ml/kg. If stool output is 10-12 stools per day or 10-20 grams/kg per day, then no changes should be made to the enteral rate. If stool output is more than 12 stools per day or greater than 20 grams/kg, feedings should be reduced to previously tolerated rate or temporarily held for 8 hours then restarted at 75% of previously tolerated rate. Ostomy output can be assessed in a similar way. If output is 2-3 grams/kg, no changes in tube feeding plan should be made. If output is less than this, the tube feeding can be advanced by 10-20 ml/kg. If the ostomy output is above this, then no change should be made to the tube feeding plan. Reducing substances should also be monitored daily. A finding of greater than 1% indicates the need to reduce or hold feedings due to malabsorption.

Common complications

The most common medical complication for children receiving long term PN is line sepsis. Staphylococcus is the most common pathogen. Line sepsis occurs due a number of reasons including frequent needle sticks into the line or bacterial translocation from the gut. Another common complication is thrombosis formation, which is very dangerous and can lead to death. Long term PN can also lead to cholestatic liver disease. This is thought to be due to lack of stimulation in the GI tract from enteral nutrition. Lack of enteral nutrition can also cause problems with the gall bladder because it is not being stimulated. This can prevent the gall bladder from being emptied leading to gallstones.

Bacterial overgrowth

Bacterial overgrowth occurs when excessive amounts of bacteria from the colon migrate into the small intestine. This can typically occur when the ileocecal valve has been removed during surgical resection of the small intestine. Symptoms of bacterial overgrowth can include diarrhea, abdominal pain, excessive gas production and bloating. Bacterial overgrowth can contribute to the overall malabsorption that is present in SBS. Specifically, carbohydrate malabsorption occurs due to bacterial action on carbohydrate as it enters the small intestine. This causes the excessive gas. The bacteria present also causes a decrease in hydrolase activity at the brush border and causes further mucosal injury. Fat malabsorption also occurs because the presence of bacteria in the small intestine affects bile salt metabolism. Many children with SBS will receive cycled antibiotics such as Flagyl every 1-2 weeks to help control bacteria.

Celiac Disease

Celiac Disease is an autoimmune disorder of the small intestine causing a lifelong intolerance to gluten. Gluten is a type of protein that includes gliadin and is found in barley, wheat and rye. Clinical symptoms of Celiac Disease include constipation or diarrhea, abdominal pain and distention, vomiting, malodorous stools, skin rash, and chronic fatigue. It can also cause weight loss and failure to thrive in infants and young children. Other symptoms can include anemia, behavioral changes, osteopenia and bone pain. Celiac Disease is often associated with other autoimmune disorders such as type 1 diabetes. Biopsy of the small intestine is the best diagnostic tool. A follow up biopsy after dietary changes have been made should be performed to monitor for recovery of the mucosa of the small intestine.

Nutrition intervention

A child that needs to follow a gluten free diet because of Celiac Disease should have family support behind him or her. The foods the child is allowed should be emphasizes rather than the foods not allowed. A readily available list is helpful as well as a designated snack area. It is recommended that the entire family follow a gluten free diet while at home. The main nutrition intervention is a gluten free, gliadin free diet. Wheat, barley, and rye should be eliminated from the diet as well as oats. Although oats do not contain gluten, they may be harmful to the mucosa. The gluten free diet is very challenging especially for foods eaten outside the home such as school or restaurants. If the diet is strictly adhered to, symptoms should abate and mucosal healing will occur.

Grains and flours can include arrowroot starch, potato starch, legume flour, rice flour, soy flour, cornmeal, cornstarch or tapioca starch. Breads should be made from allowed flours or a commercial gluten free baking mix. Cereals can be made from corn, rice or hominy. Pastas should be rice pasta, bean pasta or commercial gluten free pasta that are also low in protein. For crackers and snack type foods, rice crackers, cornmeal tortillas, crackers from appropriate flours and potato chips are available. Labels should be carefully inspected for appropriateness. Gluten is hidden in many food additives and ingredients such as malt flavoring, distilled vinegar, or modified starch. Gluten can also be found in candy, sauces, salad dressings, gravy, soups, and vegetables in sauces. Frequent and consistent reading of food labels is required including those of previously safe foods as ingredients may change at any time.

Food hypersensitivity and food intolerance

A food hypersensitivity is when an immune reaction occurs after consuming a certain food or food additive. These can be IgE (immunoglobulin E) mediated reactions where the response occurs within 1 hour. They can also be non-IgE mediated such as gluten sensitive enteropathy. The most common food hypersensitivities in children are milk, eggs, wheat, peanut, and soybean. The most common in older children and adults are fish, shellfish, peanuts and nuts. Food intolerance is an abnormal response to a food but is not immune related. These can be due to food additives such as dyes, preservatives or sweeteners. This can also be due to various types of unintentional toxins such as oxalates, staphylococcus aureus, and algal toxins such as saxitoxin found in shellfish. Food intolerance can also be a result of structural abnormalities in the GI tract such as hiatal hernia, congenital reasons such as sucrase deficiency, or acquired intolerance such as secondary lactose intolerance.

Manifestation

Three common ways that food hypersensitivities can manifest are gastrointestinal (GI), cutaneous, and respiratory. The reactions can be further divided into IgE and non-IgE mediated reactions. For GI- IgE mediated reaction, the typical response may be itching around the mouth and oral area, throat tightness, nausea, vomiting, diarrhea and possibly colic in infancy. Non- IgE mediated reaction include food related enterocolitis 1-2 hours after eating with symptoms of diarrhea or vomiting, food induced proctocolitis where symptoms include bloody stools 1-3 hours after eating or Celiac Disease. Allergic eosinophilic esophagitis would be considered a mixed reaction. For cutaneous IgE mediated reactions, symptoms would include acute hives or generalized flushing. Non-IgE mediated reactions would include contact hypersensitivity, contact irritation or chronic dermatitis. Respiratory IgE mediated reactions would include rhinoconjunctivitis or laryngeal edema. Asthma would be considered a mixed reaction.

Evaluating for food hypersensitivity

The medical history should include what food is suspected in causing the reaction and how much was consumed. The type of symptoms experienced and the amount of time between when the food was eaten and symptoms presented should be noted. If the symptoms happened quickly (i.e. minutes to hours), then a food hypersensitivity is likely. Other areas to be explores would be if this type of reaction happened before with the same food and how long it has been since the last reaction. The physical exam would look for symptoms such as atopic dermatitis, rash, hives, asthma, or allergic rhinitis. Anthropometric information should be obtained and overall assessment of nutritional status should be noted. The diet diary is a tool for families to keep a detailed food diary that records all foods, snacks and beverages consumed with portion sizes and times consumed. Any symptoms that present and the timing should be documented in the diary. The diary should also include all medications or vitamins taken, brand names of foods, and any recipes used.

Prick skin testing

If food hypersensitivity is suspected, PST will help to determine what food is responsible. Food extracts are applied by needle prick then the size of the wheal or welt is measured to determine if a positive reaction occurred. A PST is positive if the size of the wheal is 3 mm more than the control and indicates that there was an IgE present for that food but it does not necessarily mean the child will have a clinical reaction. Infants less than a year may not have a positive PST due to low levels of IgE but can still have an IgE mediated allergy. Children less than 2 may have a smaller wheal than older kids and may in fact have an IgE mediated allergy. RAST is a radioallergosorbent test. This is an in vitro assay that checks for serum specific IgE antibodies. This test will show whether specific levels of IgE are present for individual food items and the likelihood that the child will have a clinical reaction if challenged with that food.

Elimination diets

Elimination diet is when certain foods are removed from the diet based on results of the prick skin test (PST) or RAST. Foods can also be eliminated based on the patient's history or food diary. The elimination diet is usually followed by a food challenge. If symptoms are present but lab tests and history do not identify food allergens, a strict allergen elimination diet should be initiated. This diet should be used for less than 6 weeks as it can lead to nutritional deficiencies. Infants less than 4 months will typically be fed a casein hydrolysate formula such as Nutramigen or Alimentum, or an amino acid based formula such as Neocate or EleCare. Infants 4-8 months will receive the formula plus rice cereal and pears. Children 9-24 months will receive the aforementioned foods plus rice, squash and lamb. Children over 2 years will receive the aforementioned diet plus lettuce, potato, safflower oil, tea, sugar and possibly Neocate One Plus. Rice milk is sometimes used for older children not consuming any formula.

Food challenges

Open and single-blinded

An open food challenge is where the patient consumes a serving of the food thought to be causing the reaction. The response is noted. Good patients for this type of challenge are those with a negative skin test or those who have been avoiding the food on their own terms (i.e. eggs are avoided but foods containing eggs are not). A single-blinded food challenge is where a child and parent do not know what food is being challenged but the clinician knows. This can be done in an office setting and medical supervision should be present in case of anaphylaxis. If the challenge is positive, the double-blinded placebo-controlled (DBPC) food challenge should be conducted.

Double-blinded placebo-controlled

The double-blinded placebo-controlled (DBPC) food challenge is considered the gold standard for documenting food hypersensitivities. The child, parent and clinician do not know what food is being challenged. It is the most objective and accurate of all types of food challenges. A dry, powdered form of the food is used such as powdered milk or powdered eggs. A starting dose of the food approximately $1/20^{th}$ of the portion is given to the child. The dose is doubled every 10-60 minutes. Reaction to the challenge is closely monitored. If no reactivity is seen when 10 grams of the food has been provided, then an open food challenge can be conducted to further observe for any symptoms. If no reaction occurs, then the food hypersensitivity to that particular food is considered negative.

Food allergies

Comprehensive diet education is fundamentally important to achieving good compliance and a well balanced diet. Cooking from scratch and trying to avoid commercially prepared foods as much as possible are the best ways to control food allergies and to prevent ingestion of an allergen by accident. A single food allergy such as peanut will not compromise the integrity if the diet. Multiple allergens such as egg, wheat, milk and soy will

- 63 -

affect the integrity of the diet. The family needs to understand how various micro and macro nutrient needs can be met. These types of allergens are often hidden in other foods. For example, modified food starch could contain wheat or soy among other possibilities. Label reading must become a habit. Ingredients in previously safe products can change without any notice. Families need to be educated on the key words that pertain to that particular food or foods the child is allergic to. There are many books available and the Food Allergy and Anaphylaxis Network is also a great resource.

Milk protein hypersensitivity

Symptoms of milk protein hypersensitivity include vomiting, diarrhea, blood in stools, and abdominal pain. Symptoms can also be cutaneous in nature with eczema or rash. Respiratory symptoms such as wheezing or cough are possible but anaphylactic shock is rare. Infants with milk protein hypersensitivity should be changed to a formula with hydrolyzed protein such as Nutramigen, Pregestimil or Alimentum. A soy formula is not a good option as 30-50% of these infants will also be reactive to soy unless the infant has had a negative test for soy. If the hydrolyzed protein formula is not tolerated, an amino acid based formula such as Neocate or EleCare should be used. These formulas should be continued for as long as possible and not stopped when the infant turns a year. The child will be more likely to receive adequate calcium, phosphorus, vitamin D, vitamin B12 and other B vitamins.

Milk alternatives

Children will often outgrow their milk protein hypersensitivity by age 3. Many parents will inquire about using goat's milk, however, this is not an appropriate option because the infant will likely react to similar components in goat's milk. Additionally, goat's milk has a high renal solute load and is deficient in folate, iron, and vitamins A, C, and D. Parents will also inquire about using soy beverages. One fortified with vitamin D can be used but soymilk lacks the added methionine found in soy infant formulas that can improve nitrogen utilization. Rice milk is usually fortified with calcium and vitamin D but is low in protein. Parents will need to be educated about increasing protein sources in the child's diet.

<u>Egg sensitivity</u>

The protein provided form egg sources can easily be substituted with other protein sources. The main issue is with the use of eggs in many products including baked goods, breads, salad dressings and many other commercially prepared foods. Families need to learn how to adapt recipes using substitute ingredients that will be able to provide the binding and leavening properties that eggs do. Care must be taken with egg substitute, as they will likely include egg whites. An egg free powdered substitute is available called Egg Replacer. Other substitutes include using combinations of baking powder or soda, vinegar, yeast, gelatin, tofu or apricot puree in recipes. Cookbooks are available to assist with making these substitutions.

<u>Soy and wheat hypersensitivities</u>

Soy hypersensitivity typically involves the protein portion of soy. Those who are sensitive to soy are usually not sensitive to soybean oil or soy lecithin as the protein is removed during processing. Careful label reading is required as soy is present in many processed grain products, frozen dinners, sauces, salad dressings and many other items. It is frequently found in Asian food. Wheat hypersensitivity is one of the most difficult to implement, as wheat is difficult to remove from the diet. Wheat is found in a large variety of cereals, breads, pasta, soup, sauces, and even processed meats. Specialty products using an appropriate substitute flour such as arrowroot, corn, potato, rice, or rye can be found in some grocery stores, health food stores or ca n be ordered online. Gluten free products are an option but labels need to be monitored to make sure the product does not contain any other potential allergen if the child has multiple allergies. Possible deficiencies with wheat hypersensitivity can include niacin, thiamin, riboflavin, selenium, chromium and possibly iron.

NCHS growth charts

The NCHS growth charts are the most commonly used growth charts to track growth data for infants through age 20. Measurements are plotted and careful interpretation is needed. Possible clinical significance of the following parameters:

- Weight less than 10% for age- possible weight deficit requiring full evaluation
- Weight greater than 90% for age- possible weight excess requiring full evaluation

- Weight as percent of standard- weight can also be interpreted using a percentage of standard weight (or actual weight compared to weight at the 50% for age). Weight greater than 120% of standard indicates excess weight, weight between 80-90% of standard indicates marginal deficiency, weight between 60-80% of standard indicates moderate deficiency and weight less than 60% of standard indicates severe deficiency.
- Length less than 5% for age- possible severe deficit
- Length 5-10% for age- possible deficit that requires further investigation into growth velocity, overall growth pattern, and stature of parents. Other factors to consider include inaccurate measurement or incorrect technique. Length can indicate growth failure/stunting, chronic malnutrition or under nutrition.
- Head circumference less than 5% for age- can indicate chronic under nutrition in-utero or early in infancy. Length followed by weight is affected by poor nutrition before head circumference. Any excesses in head circumference velocity can indicate possible medical issues such as hydrocephalus and should be investigated immediately.
- Weight for length at 50%- indicates weight is appropriately proportioned to length or height. Greater than 90% would indicate over nutrition and less than 10% would indicate under nutrition.

Signs of deficiency

Possible signs of deficiency are as follows:
- Protein- generalized edema, thin skin, hair that is easily plucked.
- Vitamin A- retinal degeneration, Bitot's spots (gray, yellow or white spots on the whites of the eyes), keratomalacia (softening of the cornea), hyperkeratosis, night blindness, decreased immune function.
- Vitamin D- rickets, rachitic rosary, enlargement of the costochondral junction, bowed legs, osteomalacia, increased parathyroid hormone, decreased serum phosphorus, decreased serum calcium.
- Vitamin E- there is often no early signs of deficiency; later signs can include hemolytic anemia, cerebellar ataxia.
- Vitamin K- prolonged clotting, easily bruised, bleeds easily, ecchymoses

- Copper- anemia, pallor, neutropeni; count

- Fluoride- cavities, poor dentition, os

- Iron- anemia, irritability, pallor, leth

- Zinc- growth failure, poor wound he. loss of hair, diarrhea, taste changes, phosphorus

- Vitamin C- scurvy, poor wound heali fatigue, bone and muscle aches.

- Vitamin B12- megaloblastic anemia (numbness or tingling in the hands an paranoia, confusion or dementia, fatig ....cath, bleeding gums, sore mouth

- Folate- megaloblastic anemia, neural tube defects, increased homocysteine levels, stomatitis, glossitis, fatigue, weakness, decreased appetite

- Niacin- pellagra (dermatitis, diarrhea, dementia, death), cheilosis, inflammation of the mucous membranes, bright red tongue, glossitis, stomatitis, nausea, weakness

- Riboflavin- angular stomatitis, cheilosis, bright red, sore tongue, photophobia

- Thiamin- glossitis, beriberi, edema, cardiac failure, tachycardia, congestive heart failure, sensory impairment, peripheral neuropathy, lower extremity weakness, mental confusion, disorientation

(partially obscured vertical text: and appreciate cultural, ethnic ... this with the delivery of op... plan. Certain behavior... eye contact in som... cultures may ...)

Administration Considerations

Cultural sensitivity and cultural competence

Cultural sensitivity is the awareness a person has about their own beliefs, customs, and values along with those of various cultural, ethnic, or religious groups. Cultural competence is the ability to work effectively with people from other cultural, ethnic or religious backgrounds, to with those who speak a different language. In nutrition counseling, cultural sensitivity is essential because any preconceived thoughts, ideas or biases belonging to the practitioner need to be set aside in order to deliver optimal nutrition care. Cultural competence is also essential in that practitioners need to not only recognize, understand,

...r religious differences but must also find a way to balance
...imal nutritional care and encouraging compliance to the care
...s may have different meanings in different cultures such as making
...e cultures is viewed as rude, whereas not making eye contact in other
...e considered rude.

Developing cultural competence

First, the RD should examine his or her own attitudes and beliefs towards other cultures, especially those that will be a part of routing practice. Second, the RD should try to learn about other cultures including those he or she will be working with. This can be accomplished by reading books, attending seminars, using self-study guides, using the Internet, or talking with people who are a part of the culture being studied. It is especially important to understand eating patterns, typical food preferences, food preparation techniques, and food storage of other cultures. Once the knowledge base of other cultures has been expanded, the RD can begin to develop skills to address various issues that arise during nutrition assessment and counseling of various cultures. Utilizing a variety of options and interventions can help with achieving success. Another idea to increase cultural competence is to get involved with the community by attending cultural events or celebrations, by shopping at ethnic markets or by traveling to other countries. Becoming culturally competent can help the RD to interpret patient behavior more accurately.

Cultural aspects

Breastfeeding

Breastfeeding throughout the first year is a goal for many cultures. Breastfeeding practices can be very different between different cultural groups. Different cultures have their own ideas about what the maternal diet should consist of or for improving breast milk production. Some cultures believe colostrum should not be given to infants. Some cultures view breastfeeding as negative or inappropriate and do not provide appropriate support to a mom trying to nurse her baby, or the woman feels uncomfortable nursing in front of certain people. Ways to address different cultural considerations are by providing culturally sensitive breastfeeding support and education, try to increase the confidence of the lactating mom, encourage family involvement, and provide appropriate role models for the lactating mom. Also, food choices within the culture should be reviewed and the most nutrient dense foods should be encouraged.

<u>Feeding practices</u>

Infant feeding practices can vary between different cultures and ethnicities. Cultural sensitivity is important when assessing these factors. Some cultures start solids early in infancy and other cultures delay the introduction believing the infant will not tolerate the solids. Weaning practices also vary among cultures. Some cultures give sugar water in the bottle, which can cause dental caries while others give high amounts of tap water, which can cause fluorosis or hyponatremia. Some cultures such as the Asian culture often use a bottle at bedtime to help with sleep. Many moms who participate in the WIC program add food to bottles or use other types of liquids beside formula in bottles. Culturally sensitive education would involve reviewing feeding practices and the mom's cultural beliefs, encouraging selection of high nutrient dense foods within cultural norms and use appropriate education tools such as pictures or food models to make a point. The use of a language interpreter is greatly recommended when trying to educate to a person speaking a different language.

Healthy eating habits and regular exercise is a goal for all cultures but is especially important to teach to children and adolescents to help reduce their risk of developing chronic diseases. Obesity as is type 2 diabetes is on the rise especially within the American Indian, African American and Hispanic children and adolescents in America. Intake of fresh fruits and vegetables is inconsistent between cultures. In working with this population, culturally appropriate and nutrient dense foods should be encouraged while the less nutritious types of Western foods should be discouraged. Nutrition screening is important to identify at risk children and adolescents and the introduction of preventative health programs is invaluable. Parents and family should be included in education and counseling.

Federally funded food programs

- The Food Stamp Program is program designed to help low-income families buy food they need to stay healthy.

- National School Lunch Program is a program that provides free or reduced cost lunches for children whose family meets the income guidelines. The lunch will provide 1/3 of the RDA for key nutrients but must also provide less than 30% of the calories from fat
- School Breakfast Program is a program that provides free or reduced cost breakfasts to children. The breakfast must provide ¼ of the RDA for key nutrients and must also provide less than 30% of the calories from fat
- WIC is the Special Supplemental Nutrition Program for Women, Infants, and Children. This program is an attempt to improve the nutritional status of low-income pregnant or lactating women, infants and children under the age of 5. This is a no cost program for the participants and provides food packages that may include milk, cereal, cheese, or infant formula. Participants also receive nutrition education and breast feeding instruction.

Feeding

Breastfeeding

Benefits for preterm infants

Breast milk is the best way to feed any infant but is particularly beneficial to preterm infants. Breast milk contains antibodies, anti infective factors and enzymes important to developing immune and GI systems. Breast milk contains arachidonic acid and docosahexaenoic acid, which is beneficial in retinal and brain development. The nutrients in breast milk are easily absorbed and its nutrient composition is unique. Enteral feedings using breast milk are better tolerated and babies are more likely to reach full enteral feedings sooner than those fed with preterm formulas. The risk for necrotizing enterocolitis (NEC) is decreased with breast milk. The ability of a new mom to provide breast milk to a preterm infant allows for maternal infant bond to be established and provides the mom a way to focus during the ups and downs of a NICU stay.

Newborn period

The most important factor in successful breastfeeding is the support the mom receives from the father of the baby, her family and medical staff. Initial breastfeeding should occur quickly after delivery within 1 hour of life if possible. The baby is alert at this time and should be able to latch on and begin sucking. Proper positioning is important so the mom is comfortable. Pillows should be used. Changing positions with each breastfeeding session is recommended to vary the pressure on the mom's breast as well as allowing for complete emptying of milk ducts. To help the baby latch, the mom should stimulate the rooting reflex by gently touching the baby's cheek closest to the breast the baby will feed from. Once the baby's mouth is open wide, proper latching should occur with the lower lip turned out, the tongue under the nipple with the majority of the areola in the baby's mouth. The initial quick sucking is followed by a more gentle such and swallow that will stimulate the milk ejection reflex.

Nutrient composition

As beneficial as breast milk is however, its nutrient composition is not appropriate to meet the needs for rapid growth in a preterm infant. Preterm breast milk does contain higher amounts of protein and sodium for the first 28 days but is still not enough to meet the increased needs. Breast milk is not adequate in calories, calcium, phosphorus, vitamin D and iron for preterm infants. Human milk fortifiers need to be added to the breast milk to improve the nutritional composition. There are several human milk fortifiers available for hospital use in powder and liquid form. One packet of powder added to 25 cc of breast milk provides approximately 24 kcal/ounce. If a low iron fortifier is used, iron will need to be supplemented. Sodium supplementation is sometimes required with the use of fortified breast milk.

Feeding time table

The newborn baby should breastfeed every 2-3 hours 8-12 times per day to establish the mom's milk supply. The first breast should be emptied completely so the baby gets the benefits of hind milk. Breasts should be alternated at each feeding. The mom should observe the baby for active sucking to determine the length of the breastfeeding session. A newborn that is receiving enough breastmilk will have 6-8 wet diapers per day (4-5 wet, heavy disposables). The infant will be feeding the appropriate number of times per day and will completely empty the breast. This is typically accomplished in 15-20 minutes. The baby will be healthy appearing, will appear satisfied after nursing and will be gaining approximately 1 ounce per day. The baby will stool frequently at least 3 times per day or with every feeding.

Supplements

The nutrients that should be supplemented in a breastfed baby are:

- Vitamin K- all newborns need to receive intramuscular vitamin k at 0.5-1 mg to prevent hemorrhagic disease of the newborn
- Vitamin D- this needs to be supplemented at 200 IU per day to meet the RDA to prevent rickets. This is especially important when the maternal diet is deficient, the mom or baby is kept covered for religious reasons, is dark skinned, whose mom is lactose intolerant or vegan should be supplemented.
- Fluoride- this mineral does not transfer through breast milk. Exclusively breastfed infants should receive supplementation of 0.25 mg/day starting at 6 months. This helps with tooth development and the prevention of caries.
- Iron- the bioavailability of iron in breast milk is high but supplementation should start at around 6 months of age to prevent iron deficiency anemia. Iron stores in the newborn typically last from 4-6 months.
- Vitamin B12- infants of lactating moms who follow a strict vegan diet and do not take vitamin B12 supplements should receive 0.3-0.5 mcg per day to prevent deficiency

Pumping and storage

Lactating moms of sick infants or who are unable to physically nurse for some reason need to pump their breast milk until the infant is able to nurse. Pumping can be done manually by hand, by a hand held pump or by an electric breast pump. Pumping should typically occur 8-12 times per day to establish and maintain the mom's milk supply. If the infant is not able to breast feed at all or is unable to use the breast milk that is pumped, proper storage techniques should be followed. Mature breast milk can be stored at room temperature for up to 24 hours and up to 8 days in the refrigerator. Freezing milk is an option for longer storage. Storage in a freezer that is within the refrigerator is 2 weeks, 3-4 months in a freezer that is in a separate compartment than the refrigerator, and 6 months in a deep freezer. Breast milk should be frozen in small portions to minimize waster. Glass containers are preferred but polypropylene plastic can also be used.

<u>Weaning from the breast</u>

The American Academy of Pediatrics recommends breast feeding for a year then longer if both the mother and child want to. Weaning from the breast can occur with transitioning to either a cup or a bottle if less than a year of age. Self-weaning can also occur as the infant gradually increases the intake of solid food. At around a year of age, 25% of the infant's calories should be from breast milk with the remainder from solid food. For children who are bottle-feeding, after a year whole milk can replace formula and can be provided in a cup. 12-16 ounces per day is required to meet calcium requirements. If the child has difficulty giving up the bottle, weaning can be delayed until 18-24 months if the child is held while given the bottle. The child should not be allowed frequent access to the bottle, be allowed to walk around with the bottle or go to sleep with it. Substituting water for any other liquid in the bottle can be helpful.

Formulas

If breast milk is not an option, formulas for preterm infants are available and are specially designed to meet the increased nutritional requirements of preterm infants. Preterm formulas are available as ready to feed liquid in calorie concentration of 20 kcal/ounce and 24 kcal/ounce. The carbohydrate content is approximately 50% glucose polymers and 50% lactose for improved digestion. Lactase activity is present but in lower levels than term infants. The fat source is 40-50% medium chain triglycerides to promote better absorption by the preterm infant. Pancreatic lipase and bile salts are not fully present yet. The protein source is 60/40 whey to casein ratio. This ratio provides more cysteine and less tyrosine and phenylalanine for better tolerance. Calcium and phosphorus content is appropriate to meet the increased needs for bone mineralization and to promote accretion rates similar to in utero rates. The sodium, potassium and chloride content are higher than in term formulas. Vitamins and minerals are added in increased levels to meet the unique requirements of a growing preterm infant. These formulas are iron fortified.

<u>Transitional formulas</u>

Transitional formulas such as Similac NeoSure Advance or Enfamil EnfaCare Lipil are designed to meet the increased nutritional requirements of a preterm infant at discharge. The nutrient composition falls between that of a term formula and a preterm formula.

Preterm infants can be transitioned to this type of formula at approximately 1.8 kg prior to discharge. Research has found transitional formulas to be particularly beneficial to infants with a birth weight less than 1.25 kg by improving bone mineralization, improving linear and head circumference growth as well as overall improved weight gain after discharge. The formula contains a mix of glucose polymers and lactose for improved tolerance. The fat composition is approximately 25% as medium chain triglycerides and the remainder as long chain fats. The protein source is a 50/50 ratio of whey to casein. Vitamins and minerals including calcium, phosphorus and iron are provided at levels appropriate for a growing preterm infant. Transitional formulas are available as 22 kcal/ounce liquid and as powder that can be concentrated to the desired calorie concentration.

Appropriate use

Standard infant formulas are not appropriate for use in preterm infants during the neonatal period. This type of formula is nutritionally inadequate to meet the increased needs for rapid growth and development. The carbohydrate source in term formulas is lactose and the fat is typically long chain. Preterm infants may not tolerate this type of formula because lactase and pancreatic lipase activity is reduced. Standard infant formulas may be an option for a larger preterm infant who is consistently gaining greater than 30 grams per day and consuming at least 180 ml/kg of formula. Elemental formulas are also nutritionally inadequate for a preterm infant. In certain cases such as recovery from GI issues, however, an elemental formula may be indicated and unavoidable. If an elemental formula is required, the infant will need to be transitioned appropriately to a preterm formulation. Soy formulas are not indicated for preterm infants less than 1.8 kg. Phytates present in soy formula bind the phosphorus and increase the risk for osteopenia. Decreased growth has also been demonstrated in preterm infants receiving soy formula.

Standard cow's infant formula

Standard cow's milk formula is the appropriate substitution for breast milk if this is not available. The protein source is a combination of casein and whey. Fat is a blend of vegetable fats including saturated and polyunsaturated fats. Fat contributes 40-50% of total calories, which is important for developing brains. Arachidonic acid (AA) and docosahexaenoic acid (DHA) have been added to many infant formulas to reportedly assist with brain and eye development. The carbohydrate source is lactose. Lactose free formulas

- 74 -

are available even though the actual incidence of primary lactose intolerance remains rare. A lactose free formula may be indicated following a gastrointestinal upset. Standard formulas are iron fortified. Low iron formulas are available but not recommended by the American Academy of Pediatrics due to the risk and complications of iron deficiency anemia in infants.

Infant formulas for children older than 1 year

Children older than a year have multiple options available for enteral nutrition. Infant formulas can be continued up to age 4 in certain cases. Infant formulas have a lower renal solute load than other options and changing to a pediatric formulation is sometimes difficult to do because of tolerance issues. Other options include pediatric polymeric formulas. These formulas are typically 1 calorie per ml and are designed for children between 1 and 11 years old. The formulas are isotonic, lactose free and some contain fiber. Volume needed to meet the RDA for vitamins and minerals is approximately 1000-1100 ml per day. For children over 10, either a pediatric, adult or combination of both can be used. Nutrient requirements should be considered and calculated carefully to ensure micronutrient requirements such as calcium are being met.

Soy formulas

Soy formulas were introduced during the 1960's for infants who could not digest cow's milk protein. Soy formulas are indicated for galactosemia. Soy formulas can be used for infants of vegetarian parents. They are often used for infant's with cow's milk protein allergy, however, 50-60% of infants with an allergy to cow's milk protein are also allergic to soy. Soy formulas contain higher amounts of protein because the protein quality is lower than that of cow's milk. Methionine, carnitine and taurine are added. Soy formulas are lactose free and many arc also sucrose and corn free. Phytates present in soy formula bind with iron, calcium, phosphorus and zinc; therefore, additional amounts of these nutrients are added to ensure adequate absorption.

Protein hydrolysate and amino acid based

Protein hydrolysate formulas are hypoallergenic formulas for use with infants with cow's milk protein allergy, soy allergy or malabsorption. The protein source is typically casein hydrolysate. The carbohydrate sources can vary and may include corn syrup solids, modified cornstarch, dextrose or sucrose. The fat blend can also vary from long chains to a mix of long chain and medium chain triglycerides. Protein hydrolysate formulas are more expensive than cow's milk formulas and the decision to use should be carefully considered. Amino acids based formulas are designed for infants with severe protein sensitivity. These infants cannot even tolerate protein hydrolysate. These are also used for infants with severe gastroesophageal reflux and eosinophilic esophagitis. Amino acid based formulas are extremely costly and are not always covered by WIC or insurance.

Semi-elemental, elemental, and calorically dense formulas

Semi-elemental formulas contain hydrolyzed protein in the form of peptides and amino acids. The fat source is a combination of long chain and medium chain triglycerides. The osmolality is low to moderate depending upon the product. Semi elemental formulas can be used with liver disease, inflammatory bowel disease, diarrhea or steatorrhea, and allergy to soy or cow's milk. Elemental formulas contain free amino acids, are low in fat, lactose free with a high osmolality. This type of product may be indicated for severe allergies, chylothorax, HIV, intestinal fistula or malabsorption. Calorically dense formulas contain intact protein, are lactose free and contain 1.5-2 calorie per ml. These can be used for children requiring fluid restriction, or with increased calorie requirements such as cystic fibrosis.

Fluid requirements

An easy and commonly accepted method for calculating fluid requirements is as follows:

- For weight less than 10 kg, use 100 ml/kg
- For weight between 10-20 kg, use 1000 ml for the first 10 kg then add 50 ml/kg for each kg over 10 kg
- For weight above 20 kg, use 1500 ml for the first 20 kg then add 20 ml/kg for each kg over 20 kg.

Signs of dehydration include decreased urine output, dry mucous membranes, and no tears when crying. Laboratory data would show an elevated hematocrit, elevated sodium and blood urea nitrogen, and increased urine specific gravity.

Caloric Concentration

Increasing the caloric concentration of infant formulas can be done in several different ways:

- By concentration- this can be accomplished by either adding less water to the liquid concentrate or by adding more powder. Concentrating infant formulas allows the ratio of protein, fat and carbohydrate to remain constant. Concentration up to 24-26 kcal/oz is generally well tolerated if advanced in increments of 2-4 kcal/oz.
- By adding modulars- this uses modular products such as fat or carbohydrate. If modular products are added to a base of 20 kcal/oz, the nutrient composition will likely become unbalanced and should be carefully calculated. The addition of carbohydrate or fat does not significantly increase the renal solute load although carbohydrate modulars will increase the osmolality. Protein content that contributes more than 16% of total calories may cause azotemia and increase the risk for dehydration.
- The last option would be a combination of the two methods to achieve the desired caloric concentration. The nutrient distribution can be more controlled.

Feeding methods

Feeding the preterm infant can occur in a number of ways.
- Breast/bottle- this is the preferred and most physiologic method, however, the infant must be at least 32-34 weeks gestation and medically stable to take any feedings by mouth. Also, the respiratory rate should be less than 60 breaths per minute to prevent aspiration. Prior to 32 weeks, nonnutritive sucking on a pacifier or finger should be used to help the infant correlate sucking and swallowing with satiety.
- Gavage feedings- are used for preterm infants less than 32 weeks gestation using a nasogastric tube. These feedings can be bolus or continuous. Gavage feedings can be used for infants who are intubated or who have neurologic impairment.
- Transpyloric feedings- are used for infants at risk for aspiration or with slower gut motility.
- Gastrostomy feedings- are used when there is a defect in the GI tract or for infants who are neurologically impaired. They can also be used for infants who are chronically ventilated.

Continuous and bolus feedings

Historically, continuous feedings have been provided to preterm infants. The reasons for this include less interruption of feedings and the ability to provide higher feeding volumes. Continuous feedings are beneficial to infants who have had feeding intolerance with bolus feedings, have a history of short gut syndrome, or are being fed post-pylorically. Extremely low birth weight infants just starting enteral nutrition may better tolerate continuous feedings. They can increase the risk for aspiration if the infant is placed in the prone position and not monitored closely but overall should lower aspiration risk. Recent studies, however, have shown that bolus feedings may be the preferred method of feeding. They are more physiologic and encourage a more normal pattern of GI hormone secretion after a feeding is given. Bolus feedings may promote gastric emptying and may trigger hunger/satiety cues. Bolus feedings have been shown to improve weight gain. Bolus feedings allow for more mobility as tubing can be disconnected after a feeding is given.

Feeding tubes

Blenderized tube feedings

Blenderized tube feedings are an option for feeding the pediatric patient but its use is not without risk. Blenderized tube feedings are a mixture of fruits, vegetables, meats and milk or formula. Carbohydrate and fat modulars are sometimes added. Water, vitamins and minerals are added to better meet fluid and nutrient requirements. This type of feeding has a high osmolality, contains residue, and may have a consistency that is difficult to run through a feeding tube, especially a small bore tube. Because these feedings are homemade and not sterile like commercial products, there is a risk of bacterial contamination. The formula is not emulsified and may separate. Blenderized formulas can only be delivered into the stomach because of tolerance issues. Families often select this type of formula if insurance denies coverage of commercially prepared formulas. It will save the family money. Close monitoring of hydration status and for nutritional deficiencies is imperative.

Nasogastric and gastrostomy

The main advantages of using a nasogastric tube is easy placement without the use of surgery. Nasogastric tube is indicated for short-term use of less than 1 month. The disadvantages include irritation to the nares, esophagus or trachea, may cause hypersensitive gag reflex, can be easily pulled out by a child and can be easily dislodged by forceful coughing. The advantages to a gastrostomy tube include greater mobility, able to use a larger bore tube with less chance of clogging, and does not obstruct airway. Certain gastrostomy tubes can be converted to a button device, which makes concealing the appliance much easier than with the tube present. The disadvantages are that this type of tube requires a procedure or surgery to place, possible leakage around the insertion site and the risk for peritonitis. A gastrostomy tube is indicated when tube feedings are expected to be needed for more than 4-6 weeks such as neurological impairment.

Continuous tube feedings

Continuous tube feedings are delivered at a steady rate using a feeding pump. Continuous tube feedings are useful in children who have not had enteral nutrition for a prolonged period or who require a slow initiation. Continuous tube feedings can be administered into the stomach and is the only method for tube feeding delivery into the small bowel, as there is no reservoir present for using other methods of delivery. Continuous tube feedings are often better tolerated than bolus feedings and may decrease the risk for aspiration. The disadvantages to continuous tube feedings are that they require more equipment and supplies and are therefore more costly. Mobility is also limited unless a portable feeding pump is used.

Bolus tube feeding

Bolus tube feeding is a method of feeding that is a convenient way to supplement oral intake. For patients who can take food and formula by mouth, it allows the child to take what he/she is able to with the remainder of the calories required given by via bolus. Pumps are generally not required as the formula is given by syringe. Mobility is generally not an issue as the child is able to move around freely. The disadvantage to bolus tube feedings is there is an increased risk for aspiration. Also, children with delayed gastric emptying or who have gastroesophageal reflux may not be able to tolerate the amount of volume in a bolus.

Intermittent tube feeding

Intermittent tube feeding delivery is the total amount of formula required for the day is divided into 5-8 feedings and is delivered using a syringe, gravity drip or a feeding pump.

The advantage to this method of feeding is that it is more physiologic and the schedule is closer to normal eating routines. It is associated with reduced costs if a feeding pump is not used and it allows for greater mobility since the child is not attached to a pump for prolonged periods. The disadvantages to intermittent delivery can include poor tolerance in critically ill children. There is an increased risk for dumping syndrome if delivered into the small bowel because there is no reservoir in the small bowel. Delivery into the stomach is recommended. There is a risk for reflux, diarrhea and emesis because a larger volume is provided. Intermittent tube feedings are a good way to gradually transition off of continuous infusion by decreasing the amount of infusion time and periods of time off the infusion.

Nocturnal tube feeding

Nocturnal tube feedings are tube feedings that are delivered at night only using a continuous infusion via feeding pump. The advantage to nocturnal tube feedings is that oral intake can be provided during the day and whatever calories need to be supplemented can be given at night. The disadvantage to nocturnal tube feedings is that the child may have difficulty sleeping fitfully because of pump noises or equipment alarms. The child may experience nausea or vomiting in the morning or may be too full to eat right away. Nocturnal tube feedings are useful in transitioning a child from continuous infusion to oral intake as this method allows for increasing oral intake while receiving the benefit of meeting nutritional requirements.

Establishing tolerance

The initial goal when starting any type of tube feeding is to establish tolerance. Isotonic formulas are preferred. It will generally take between 2-5 days to reach desired tube feeding goal. It is important to make only one change at a time of either rate or concentration as the tube feeding advances in order to detect the cause of any intolerance. Changes can be made every 8- 24 hours or by using clinical judgment. There are many different recommendations for initiating and advancing tube feedings and many institutions have their own guidelines. General guidelines for infants are to begin at 1 ml/kg/hour and advance by 1-2 ml/kg/hour. For children ages 1-6, begin at 1 ml/kg/hour and advance by 5-10 ml/hour or 1 ml/kg/hour. For children older than 7, the rate can usually start at 25 ml/hour and advance by 25 ml/hour every 8-24 hours. Bolus or intermittent feedings can begin at 5-10 ml/kg every 2-3 hours. Advancement can occur by a rate close to the starting rate and advance every 8-24 hours.

Mechanical, metabolic and growth parameters

Mechanical parameters that should be monitored include tube placement or position, site care for gastrostomy or jejunostomy tube, and nose care for nasogastric tubes. Metabolic parameters include daily intake and output and urine specific gravity. Sodium, potassium, blood urea nitrogen, creatinine, chloride, and glucose should be monitored daily until stable. Triglycerides, cholesterol, hemoglobin, hematocrit, MCV, iron, total iron binding capacity, reticulocyte count, calcium, phosphorus and magnesium should be checked initially then every week. Total protein and albumin should be checked initially then every 2 weeks. Growth parameters should include daily weights, weekly length or height, and weekly head circumference for children less than 3 years, Triceps skin fold and mid-arm muscle circumference should be checked initially then every 2-4 weeks.

GI parameters

Gastric residuals can be monitored prior to each feeding if bolus or intermittent feedings are used or every 3-4 hours if continuous infusion is used. A large gastric residual is considered to be more than 2 hours of tube feeding for continuous tube feedings or more than half the volume given at the previous feeding for intermittent or bolus. Residuals do not need to be monitored for small bowel tube feedings, as there is no reservoir in the small bowel. The level of gastric residuals should be used in conjunction with monitoring of other signs for intolerance such as an increase in abdominal girth, changes in stool pattern, color, consistency, or frequency. Gastric residuals can be elevated related to high osmolality of the formula or high fat content of the formula, which may cause delayed gastric emptying. Certain medications may also cause high gastric residuals as they may adversely affect peristalsis such as certain pain medications.

Breast milk for tube feedings

Breast milk is the optimal food for infants. Infants who are not able to nurse can still receive the benefits of breast milk through a feeding tube. Fortifiers can also be added for additional nutrition. Lactating moms need to pump and safely collect and store breast milk for their babies. Intermittent or bolus tube feeding is the preferred method of tube feeding delivery for breast milk. The use of continuous infusion tends to reduce the amount of calories delivered because the fat separates from the breast milk and sticks to the tubing. If fortifiers are added, these can also separate out. Intermittent or bolus tube feedings have a lower chance of nutrient losses. The syringe should be inverted upwards for better nutrient delivery.

Transitioning

Careful evaluation of the child should occur to ensure the child is ready to begin to transition. The issue that necessitated the use of tube feeding should be resolved or nearly resolved. The initial feeding evaluation should evaluate oral motor skills, swallow function and should assess for oral aversion. If there is any issue found, it should be addressed before transition starts. The child's nutritional status should also be optimal. Once the child is deemed ready to begin transition, the feeding schedule should be changed to accommodate oral diet. A change from continuous to nocturnal, continuous to bolus or intermittent or a combination of both methods should occur. The child needs to feel a sense of hunger. A small reduction in caloric intake of approximately 25% from tube feedings may help to stimulate appetite as well. Close monitoring of caloric intake, weights, growth, and overall progress should be followed. Provision of calories provided from tube feeding can continue to decrease as oral nutrition improves. A reasonable goal is 75% of total calories orally for the tube feeding to be stopped.

Diarrhea

Diarrhea can be caused by a number of reasons. A child who has been without enteral nutrition for a prolonged period may have gut atrophy. Hyperosmolar formulas may also cause diarrhea. The use of an isotonic formula or diluting a hyperosmolar formula may help. Medications in the syrup or elixir form often contain sorbitol, which can cause diarrhea. Medications should be reviewed thoroughly with consultation with the pediatric pharmacist for possible interventions. Tube feedings delivered too rapidly can cause diarrhea. Return to previously tolerated rate until diarrhea resolves should occur with a plan to slowly advance rate. Recent GI illness such as gastroenteritis may cause diarrhea. Bacterial contamination can also be a cause. Hang time should be limited to 8 hours for pediatric formulas prepared from powder, 2-4 hours for breast milk or infant formula, and 24 hours for ready to hang systems if nothing has been added to the container.

Parenteral nutrition

Initiating parenteral nutrition

For premature infants, PN should be started within 24 hours but ideally it should begin shortly after birth. For infants and children who are well nourished but require PN, it should be started within 3-5 days for infants and 5-7 days for children. For infants and children with compromised nutritional status or with malnutrition, PN should be started within 1-2 days. Initial laboratory data that should be monitored when PN is initiated include:

- Blood glucose- checked at least daily as glucose infusion rate increases
- Na, K, Cl, CO2- on initiation then weekly if stable
- Total protein, albumin
- Renal function- BUN, creatinine
- Serum calcium, phosphorus, magnesium
- Serum triglycerides
- Liver function tests including Alkaline phosphatase, ALT, AST, PTT
- CBS with differential, hemoglobin, hematocrit, platelets
- Urine for glucose, pH, specific gravity

Infants and children

Indications for PN in the pediatric population include any disorder where enteral nutrition is contraindicated. This would include surgical conditions such as congenital diaphragmatic hernia, certain types of enteric fistulas, gastroschisis, omphalocele, intussusception, severe short gut syndrome especially without the ileocecal valve, and tracheoesophageal fistula. Patients with chylothorax will often require PN as will those with a prolonged postoperative ileus. Patients with severe inflammatory bowel disease, necrotizing enterocolitis, or with chronic or secretory diarrhea would also be candidates. Patients with congenital heart disease where blood flow to the gut is affected should receive PN. Patients with increased metabolic needs such as burns, trauma or spies will require PN. Premature infants should start PN and critically ill patients who are not able to tolerate enteral nutrition should start PN.

Peripheral parenteral nutrition

Peripheral parenteral nutrition (PPN) is indicated for short term use of less than 2 weeks. A line is considered peripheral if the tip is located in a vein other than the superior or inferior vena cava. A peripheral vein is much more fragile than a central artery and cannot tolerate a solution with an osmolarity greater than 900 mOsm/liter. The maximum dextrose concentration that can run through a peripheral vein is 12.5%, however, the dextrose concentration will need to be lower depending upon the concentration of amino acids. It is more difficult to fully meet a child's nutritional needs with PPN. The solutions are less nutrient dense than central solutions and more volume is needed to meet nutritional needs. The calcium concentration also needs to be restricted as it may cause an extravasation injury. Complications of PPN include phlebitis and loss of access. Peripheral sites needs to be rotated every few days.

Central access for total parental nutrition

Central total parental nutrition (TPN) is indicated for children who will require PN for greater than 2 weeks or who require a volume restriction. A surgical procedure is required to place a central venous catheter (CVC). Central access is usually placed in the inferior or superior vena cava where this large artery can handle a solution with high osmolarity (more than 900 mOsm/liter). Nutritional requirements can be better met. A CVC has its tip located just outside the right atrium. CVC can be used for TPN, chemotherapy, antibiotics and blood transfusions. CVC are available with single, double and triple lumens although a neonate can only tolerate the size of a single lumen. A clean line used just for TPN is recommended. Two examples of CVS are Broviac and Hickman. Complications of a CVC include infection, thrombosis, air emboli, catheter breakage or pneumothorax.

A PICC line is a peripherally inserted central catheter that can be placed at the bedside under sterile conditions. A PICC line is usually inserted in the cephalic, basilica or median cubital vein with the tip threaded to just outside the right atrium. If the tip is not is proper position, this line should not be considered central. PICC lines can be used for up to a month. Placement should be checked if significant linear growth occurs, as the tip may not be in the proper position. Sepsis rates tend to be lower with the use of PICC lines because they are less invasive than CVC. PICC lines are less expensive than surgically placed CVC. Implantable ports include Port-a-Cath. This is a device that has a catheter surgically inserted through the neck or shoulder to the jugular, subclavian or superior vena cava. It is not as visible as other types of central access. It is appropriate for long-term use at home. Complications can include infection, pneumothorax, or thrombosis.

2 in 1 and 3 in 1 parenteral nutrition solutions

A 2 in 1 solution contains dextrose, amino acids, electrolytes, vitamins and minerals. Lipids are provided through a separate infusion. The benefit of a 2 in 1 solution is the ability to see if calcium-phosphate crystals have formed before a patient is given the solution. Infusion of a solution with crystals is extremely dangerous and can result in death. More calcium and phosphorus can be added to 2 in 1 solutions. There will be less medication interactions with the lipids separate. One disadvantage is the possibility of lipid intolerance, as lipids will be infused over a shorter period. A 3 in 1 solution is also called total nutrient admixture (TNA). This type of solution provides amino acids, lipids, dextrose, electrolytes, vitamins and minerals all in the same bag. TNA offers more convenience and is more cost effective. Temperature and pH can influence stability as can the final concentration of all macronutrients. Less calcium and phosphorus can be added and it is more difficult to see precipitates.

Dextrose

The carbohydrate source in PN solutions is dextrose monohydrate and provides 3.4 kcal/gram. Dextrose should contribute 45-60% of total calories. Dextrose is generally initiated at a glucose infusion rate (GIR) of 4-6 mg/kg/minute in infants, and 5-6 mg/kg/minute in children. A glucose infusion rate of less than 2 mg/kg/minute will not prevent ketosis. The general GIR limit for children is approximately 14 mg/kg/minute though preterm infants can tolerate up to 16 mg/kg/minute. A GIR exceeding this rate may cause hyperglycemia, fatty liver, cholestasis, overfeeding and excess CO_2 production. The GIR should be advanced slowly by 1-2 mg/kg/minute per day to help keep blood glucose levels stable and allow for insulin response to adjust. Tolerance to dextrose infusion is monitored by checking blood glucose and urine glucose. Dextrose concentration should be limited to 10-12.5% for peripheral lines and less than 30% for central. Prior to discontinuing a dextrose infusion, the GIR should be gradually weaned to prevent rebound hypoglycemia.

Amino acids

Protein should contribute 8-15% of total calories. The source of protein is crystalline amino acids and this provides 4 kcal/gram. Amino acid mixtures for pediatrics include Trophamine and Aminosyn PF. These amino acid solutions have been designed to mimic the amino acid profile of breast fed infants. In neonates, the conditionally essential amino acids are taurine, tyrosine, cysteine, and histidine. Conditionally essential means that these amino acids cannot be synthesized by the neonate. The addition of cysteine as L-cysteine hydrochloride lowers the pH of the solution and allows for greater calcium and phosphorus stability. Protein tolerance is monitored by checking BUN and ammonia levels. Acid base balance should also be monitored. Protein status is monitored by checking albumin and total protein. Prealbumin, transferrin and retinol binding protein have shorter half-lives and are therefore more sensitive to changes in protein status.

Lipid emulsions

Lipid emulsions consist of either soybean oil or a mix of soybean and safflower oils. Lipids are required to prevent essential fatty acid deficiency as well as a calorie source. Essential fatty acid deficiency can develop quickly especially in infants but can be prevented with 0.5 gram/kg per day or with 1.5 grams/kg twice per week in older children. Lipids can be provided as a 10% (1.1 kcal/ml) or 20% (2 kcal/ml) emulsion. The upper limit of fat intake is 3-4 grams per kg and should contribute 30-40% of total calories with the absolute upper limit of 60%. Contraindications to lipids, which may require omission or restriction to 0.5-1 gram/kg, are hyperbilirubinemia, sepsis, and thrombocytopenia. Fat overload can occur if lipids are not advanced slowly and are provided in amounts greater than the lipoprotein lipase activity can handle. This can cause a decrease in immune function. Lipid clearance is measure by checking serum triglyceride levels. Triglycerides should be less than 150 mg/dl if held for 2 hours before drawing or less than 200 mg/dl for a continuous infusion.

Cycled total parenteral nutrition

Cycled TPN is defined as providing TPN in a period of time that is less than 24 hours. This type of schedule is often used in the home setting as it allows for time off the infusion pump and for greater mobility. Younger infants receiving only TPN may tolerate up to 4 hours off the infusion while older children may be able to tolerate up to 6-8 hours. Concerns with this would include maintenance of fluid status and glucose levels. Cycled PN is often in used in this case to provide a window off the infusion to allow the liver to rest to possible help with cholestasis. This should not be used in infants less than 3 kg.

For infants and children who receive enteral nutrition either by eating or tube feeding in addition to TPN, the TPN can be cycled over 8-12 hours. Older children will often have their TPN cycled over 10-16 hours as they can tolerate higher fluid volumes. The amount of TPN provided can be based on the amount of calories taken enterally and the absorption of the enteral nutrition. The advantages of cycled TPN are better quality of life, providing a more physiologic feeding that helps reduce persistent insulin secretion, and may help to reduce the risk of developing cholestasis. When starting a cycled TPN regimen, the initial rate should gradually increase to the desired rate over a 2 hours period then reduced over 1-2 hours at the end of the infusion to allow glucose levels to adjust.

Trace minerals

Trace minerals that are usually added to PN solutions include zinc, copper, chromium, and manganese. These are available as separate additives or as a single mix. Selenium and iodine are also available. Additional zinc is required for preterm infants and in cases of deficiency or increased losses such as enteric fistula. Selenium is not needed for short term TPN and should be omitted with impaired renal function as it is excreted in the urine. Copper should be reduced or omitted from PN in cases of cholestasis and the patient should be followed for deficiency. Manganese should be omitted with cholestasis. Both copper and manganese are excreted through bile and any impairment in the biliary system increases the risk for toxicity. Conditions that are at risk for trace element deficiency include infants and children with malnutrition, preterm infants, burn injury, chronic diarrhea, enteric fistulas, and bile salt malabsorption.

Parenteral calcium and phosphorus requirements

The recommendations for children over 1 year of age for calcium is 0.5-1 mEq/kg and for phosphorus 0.5-1.3 mmol/kg. The most common type of calcium additive is calcium gluconate. A 10% calcium gluconate solution provides 100 mg of calcium gluconate or 10 mg elemental calcium in 1 ml. Phosphorus is added as potassium phosphate or sodium phosphate salts. Both provide 3 mmol (93 mg) pf elemental phosphorus per 1 ml. Temperature and increased pH levels as well as dextrose concentration and decreased amino acid content can limit calcium and phosphorus solubility. The order of compounding is also important and the addition of L-cysteine will increase solubility. The recommended calcium to phosphorus ratio is 1.1-1.3:1 molar ratio or 1.3:1 to 1.7:1 ratio by weight. Providing an inappropriate ratio may lead to hypercalcemia, hypercalciuria, hypophosphatemia and altered mineral homeostasis depending upon the final ratio.

Prescription

The following information is required in order to effectively write a prescription for PN:

- Name and date of birth
- Current weight or weight that will be used for dosing
- Type of access- peripheral or central
- Fluid prescription and total PN volume for the day
- Rate of infusion and number of hours it will be infused for
- Dextrose, amino acid and lipids- written in grams per volume or grams per kg or grams per day but should be clearly specified and consistent
- Amount of electrolytes- should also be clearly specified and consistent with established guidelines for the institution
- Vitamins and trace element amounts

Intravenous lipids

Intravenous fat can be started at 0.5-1 gram/kg depending upon the age of the patient and can be advanced by 0.25-0.5 grams/kg per day to desired amount. The maximum infusion rate for lipids is 0.12-0.15 grams/kg/minute. This is approximately 3-3.6 grams/kg per day. During periods of sepsis, the dose should be limited to 0.08 grams/kg/minute. Possible consequences that may occur if the maximum lipid infusion rate is exceeded include impaired lung function, decreased immune function and the risk for kernicterus if the serum bilirubin is also increased. Lipids that are part of a total nutrient admixture can be safely hung for 24 hours. For a separate lipid infusion, the hang time should be limited to 12 hours due the risk for bacteremia. The use of a 1.2 micron filter with total nutrient admixtures will help to filter large particles, precipitates, and globules of fat and provide a measure of safety.

<u>Home parenteral nutrition</u>

Children who require Home parenteral nutrition (HPN) typically require this for at least one year. For this reason, it is important for a child to have a stable home life. At least 2 adults should be trained to knowledgeably provide care and extended family support is also helpful. Safety procedures should be closely followed to prevent injury to other family members form needle sticks, etc. The home should be clean with electric power, refrigeration, phone service and a safe water supply. A home care agency with nursing support it required to assist with supplies, monitoring of laboratory data, tolerance and overall clinical condition of the child along with periodic nutrition reassessment. Appropriate medical insurance is needed to cover the costs of HPN.

Enteral nutrition

Pediatric candidates for enteral nutrition support would include the following:

- Children with caloric intake less than 80% of estimated requirements
- Lack of consistent weight gain over 3 month period
- Unexplained weight loss over 3 months or more
- Weight/length or weight/height below the 5% for age
- Children who require a prolonged length of time for feeding (4-6 hours per day or more)
- Children with significant oral aversion
- Children who are not able to properly or safely chew or swallow
- Children with malnutrition
- Children with malabsorption, short bowel syndrome, cystic fibrosis, neurological impairment or with increased calorie requirements such as burns, trauma or sepsis
- Children with esophageal obstruction or with congenital anomalies such as esophageal atresia, tracheoesophageal fistula or cleft palate

Thickening agent

Infants who have been identified by modified barium swallow as having a swallowing disorder often requires the use of a thickening agent to decrease aspiration risk. The type of thickening agent used is important to consider. A gel thickener is made from xanthan gum and does not contribute carbohydrate or calories. A powdered thickener does contribute calories as it is made from carbohydrate. The amount of additional calories added can be significant because 1 tablespoon of powder contains 15 calories. This may increase caloric intake by up to 25% that in turn may lead to rapid weight gain. Rice cereal is also used at times but it does not thicken consistently, does not blend easily and it also contributes calories. Providing adequate fluid intake is also an issue as the addition of thickening agent replaces fluid.

Starting solids

A former preterm infant should not start solid foods until a corrected age of at least 4-6 months is reached. Many former preterm infants are not developmentally ready until closer to 6 months corrected age. Signs of readiness for solid foods should be observed such as adequate head control, able to hold trunk upright and steady, and showing signs of interest in what others are eating. It should be noted that once solid foods are started and established, consumption of formula will begin to decrease which might adversely affect growth in infants who may require the additional calories. Parent and caregivers should be fully educated on appropriate feeding practices and should be discouraged form starting solids too early or adding cow's milk before a year of corrected age.

In infancy, it is recommended that the calories be distributed as approximately 7-11% from protein, 40-50% from fat and the remainder as carbohydrate. The RDA for infants 0-6 months for calories is 108 kcal/kg and 2.2 grams per kg protein. For infants 6-12 months, the RDA is 98 kcal/kg and 1.6 grams per kg protein. From birth to around 4-6 months of age, infants have an extrusion reflex that prevents them from being able to eat solid food. After this time, the extrusion reflex begins to disappear, as sufficient oral skills have developed to allow initiation of solid foods. The gag reflex is still present until approximately 7-9 months of age. The infant is able to move the food from the front of the tongue to the back in order to swallow. Around 4-6 months, the infant also starts to imitate other. The baby will show signs of readiness by opening his or her mouth when others are eating and can turn away from food when he or she is full.

<u>4-6 months</u>

At around 6 months of age, an infant is receiving approximately 80% of calories from formula or breast milk and 20% from solids. Rice cereal is typically introduced first as it is not likely to cause an allergic reaction. Barley and oatmeal can be introduced next allowing 2-3 days in between to watch for allergic reactions. Strained fruits and vegetables can be added next followed by meats. The texture should gradually increase as the infant develops oral motor skills such as side to side chewing. By 10 months of age, half of the infant's calories are from solids. By around a year of age, the infant should be able to handle soft chopped table foods that the rest of the family is enjoying. It should be noted that an infant might require multiple attempts at new foods or textures before it is accepted.

<u>Second 6 months</u>

The infant should be allowed to work on self-feeding skills as soon as his or her grasp allows. This is typically around 7 months of age. The infant should be working on self-feeding of finger foods and towards the end of the second 6 months, should be working on spoon-feeding on their own. A sippy cup should be introduced around 6-8 months of age filled with breast milk or formula. Choking hazards for young children include whole grapes, hot dogs that have not been cut up small enough, nuts, raw carrots, broccoli or cauliflower or other tough fruits or vegetables. Hard candy, gummy bears, and marshmallows are all potential choking hazards. Pretzels, chips and popcorn should also be avoided. Any cut up food should be smaller than ½ inch in diameter.

Introducing cow's milk

Infants should be fed breast milk or iron fortified formula for the first year of life. Introducing cow's milk prior to the first may cause bleeding from the GI tract. Initial iron stores at birth will last from 4-6 months. At the time iron stores are becoming depleted, iron fortified cereal is started to provide the additional iron required. Because of this occult blood loss from the GI tract, the risk for iron deficiency anemia increases. Early introduction can also increase the risk for developing cow's milk protein allergy. As the GI tract matures, the risk for allergies decreases. Early introduction may also compromise nutritional status. Often times cow's milk will replace the more nutritious breast milk or iron fortified formula. Cow's milk is not nutritionally adequate for growing infants. It is deficient in vitamin C, vitamin E, iron, and essential fatty acids. It will provide less calories overall. Additionally, the renal solute load is higher than that of formula and this will increase the risk for dehydration.

Food choices in a child's life

There are many factors that can influence food choices in young children. Family is one of the strongest influences. Food likes and dislikes are developed in the early years and often do not change into adulthood. Parents, brothers and sisters are role models for young children and often times this is not recognized by the family. For example, if parents have a strong dislike for seafood, it is unlikely that young children will be given the opportunity to develop a taste for it thus eliminating a healthful food choice based on parental bias. It is up to the parents or caregivers to provide appropriate food choices so healthy eating habits are developed. Children also close observers of parental eating habits. Children who live with someone who is constantly "dieting" or trying to lose weight may develop distorted body image, which in turn will affect future food choices. Also, many families have both parents working outside the home and meals are often from fast food restaurants or convenience foods.

<u>Media, peers and body image</u>

There are many factors that can influence food choices in young children. The media is also a significant influence on eating habits. Children are watching more hours of television nowadays and are exposed to multiple food advertisements including fast foods, candy, snack foods, etc. Foods are shaped into favorite cartoon characters. Peer influence can have a strong influence on children. Preschoolers may be more likely to try a new food if classmates are all trying it. Teens begin to treat eating with peers as more of a social activity. Children may be made fun of if food choices are not typical of what other kids eat and thus may resist previously healthy food choices. Body image is especially influential during puberty and pre-puberty. Many girls and even more and more boys may try to change their body image using unsafe methods such as restrictive diets, supplements or pills. Children may have distorted body images due in part to what they observe on television and in magazines.

<u>Promoting healthy eating habits</u>

Preschool children are often fussy, may refuse food or may not be interested in eating at times. It is up to the parent or caregiver to offer nutritious food. A variety of foods should be offered in different shapes, colors and textures. Favorite foods can be provided but new foods or foods not previously accepted should continue to be offered. Juices, soda and other beverages should be limited between meals as too much will affect appetite at meals. The environment for meals should be quiet and without distractions. Meals and snacks should be provided at fairly consistent times to allow for hunger and because preschoolers do better with routine. The child should be allowed to decide how much to eat. This helps the child listen to satiety cues. Pushing a child to eat more can lead to over eating as the child gets older. Desserts and treats should not be used as a reward for eating well as this reinforces the child's belief that desserts and sweets are better than more healthful foods.

School age children exhibit a pattern of steady growth and have established food preferences. Change can occur during this period and continued education is important to keep developing healthy eating habits. Parents or caregivers should model good, healthy eating habits. The USDA's MyPlate is useful in meal planning. A variety of foods should be offered and new foods should continue to be trailed. Foods or snacks with low nutrient density should be limited but not forbidden as this makes the food more attractive to the child. The child should be encouraged to help plan, shop and prepare meals. The child should pay attention to satiety cues. Milk should be provided with meals to help meet calcium requirements which are often low in this age group. It is also important to serve a healthy breakfast each day as this helps with attention and learning in school. Meals should be served at the table as a family and without distractions such as the television as this can lead to overeating.

Vegetarian diet

<u>Growth concerns</u>

Adults who adhere to a vegetarian diet have less of a chance of developing numerous chronic diseases such as degenerative conditions, obesity, heart disease, hypertension, diabetes and certain types of cancers. Children who follow a vegetarian diet will be laying a good foundation for future health. It is important to meet recommendations for micro and macronutrients so growth and development is not affected. Children who are vegetarians tend to have similar growth rates compared to children who are not vegetarian. However, children who are following a very restrictive diet such as macrobiotic may have some delays in growth. Adolescent girls following a vegetarian diet may experience a delayed growth spurt and the start of menses may be delayed.

Calories and protein

Consuming adequate calories for growth may be difficult for young children due to the diet being high in fiber. Infants and toddlers at the time of weaning may have a temporary drop in growth rate. Children need to consume calorically dense foods appropriate for their diet restrictions to add calories such as avocados, nuts, seeds, or olives. If the amount of fiber in the diet causes the child to feel full and not consume adequate calories for growth, the fiber content may need to be reduced by switching to refined grains or peeled fruits and vegetables. Small, frequent meals and snacks will help as well. Protein sources should be selected carefully and should be eaten throughout the day. Protein requirements for vegetarian children may be 20-30% higher than the RDA because all the protein is not of high biological value. Lacto-ovo vegetarians can include cottage cheese, yogurt, milk, eggs and other dairy products as well as vegan protein sources such as legumes, grains, soy products, meat analogues, nuts and seeds.

Calcium and vitamin D

Calcium intake of a lacto-ovo vegetarian may exceed requirements if dairy products are consumed freely. For vegan children, intake should be closely assessed as deficiency may occur. Vegetarian sources include calcium fortified soymilk or juices, dark green leafy vegetables, fortified cereals, almonds, or black strap molasses. A calcium supplement may be required. Vitamin D requirements can be met with exposure to the sun for 20-30 minutes at least twice per week. Vitamin D metabolism is affected by sunscreen, skin coloring, and time of year that can all lead to a vitamin D deficiency especially if coupled with a vegan diet. Some foods such as soy and rice milk, and cereal are fortified with vitamin D; however, a vitamin D supplement is recommended for all vegetarian children.

Iron, vitamin B12 and zinc

The potential for iron deficiency is higher for children who follow a vegetarian diet. Food sources include iron-fortified cereal, legumes, green leafy vegetables, enriched grains and dried fruits. Bioavailability from non-heme sources is approximately 10%. Iron sources should be eaten with a vitamin C source to improve absorption and an iron supplement may be needed. Vitamin B12 deficiency is a concern mainly for vegan children. Foods fortified with vitamin B12 include soymilk, meat analogues, nutritional yeast and some breakfast cereals. A vitamin B12 supplement may be needed is these foods are not eaten on a regular basis. Zinc intake is usually adequate but the presence of phytates may decrease absorption. Requirements may be 50% higher than the DRI. Sources of zinc include whole grain breads and cereals, wheat germ, pasta, soy, tofu, dairy products and legumes.

Exercise

Hydration

Exercise works the muscles, which in turn produces body heat and raises the body temperature. As the temperature increases, the body produces sweat that leads to cooling of the body as it dissipates. It is extremely important for the child or adolescent to replace fluid losses through sweat especially during hot weather. Children who have not entered puberty yet are at risk for overheating, as they do not sweat as much as adults do. This means their bodies are less able to compensate for the excess body heat. Cardiac output is less than adults and this reduces heat transfer as well. Adequate hydration before exercise is recommended. Water is best; however, sports drinks such as Gatorade may be useful for exercise greater than an hour in duration. Fruit juices and soda are not recommended as they may lead to stomach cramping.

Carbohydrates

Carbohydrate is the preferred substrate for muscles. The liver is only able to store a small amount as glycogen that can be used for quick energy for exercise. For longer duration activities such as long distance running or cycling, the body will first use its glycogen stores followed by its own fat stores burned for energy. This occurs after 30-45 minutes of intense exercise. The recommendation for how much carbohydrate to eat depends on the time available. For 1 hour before intense exercise, a snack of 15-20 grams is needed. For 2-4 hours before, 30-40 grams is recommended. For 4-5 hours before, 50-60 grams is recommended. Fat intake should be low to moderate. After the event, glycogen stores in the muscle needs to be repleted. This can be accomplished by drinking a high carbohydrate drink then consuming a carbohydrate containing meal.

Puree diet

A puree diet is indicated for children who have difficulty chewing or swallowing. This type of diet may be used in conditions such as severe mental retardation or developmental delay, neurological impairment or conditions affecting the anatomy of the mouth or esophagus. Foods that are already pureed or strained can be used. A food processor or blender can also be utilized to prepare foods at the right consistency. Liquids such as broths, milk or gravy can be added while being processed. Pureeing individual foods separately is more attractive than pureeing all foods together. Butter, honey, sugar, cream, or gravy can be added to increase caloric content. Thickener may need to be added if the child has been identified as having issues with thin liquids. This diet can be nutritionally complete. A vitamin and mineral supplement may be indicated if a variety of foods are not consumed. An oral supplement to add calories may be needed if maintaining weight is difficult.

Practice Test

Practice Questions

1. Which of the following risk factors is most likely to be associated with being overweight?
    a. Autistic disorder
    b. Seizure disorder
    c. Prader-Willi syndrome
    d. Congenital heart disease

2. What is the percentile for body mass index on the NCHS growth curves that is considered overweight in children?
    a. 75%
    b. 85%
    c. 90%
    d. 95%

3. Which method of data collection is most likely to underreport dietary intake?
    a. 24-hour recall
    b. Diet history
    c. 7-day food record
    d. Food frequency

4. Which of the following are the most commonly seen symptoms of a cow's milk allergy in an infant? (Choose 4 options)
    a. Constipation
    b. Atopic dermatitisc
    c. Asthma
    d Anaphylaxis
    e. Blood in the stool
    f. Vomiting

5. Which of the following foods are not allowed on a wheat-free diet? (Choose 4 options)
    a. Couscous
    b. Buckwheat
    c. Quinoa
    d. Rye
    e. Bulgur
    f. Farina
    g. Arrowroot
    h. Semolina

6. All of the following are absolute contraindications to breastfeeding EXCEPT
   a. active use of illicit drugs.
   b. use of chemotherapy agents.
   c. antiretroviral medications.
   d. alcohol.

7. A 10-year-old boy has a history of inflammatory bowel disease (IBD). He is taking sulfasalazine as part of his treatment plan. What nutrient may be adversely affected by the use of sulfasalazine?
   a. Niacin
   b. Folic acid
   c. Vitamin A
   d. Zinc

8. Which of the following is the most important diagnostic indicator for a teenage patient suspected of having anorexia nervosa?
   a. Significant fear of gaining weight
   b. Absence of at least 3 consecutive menstrual cycles
   c. Body weight that is less than 85% of expected weight
   d. Body mass index of 18 kg/m²

9. Which of the following best describes the average growth rate of a preschool age child?
   a. 5-6 cm and 4-6 kg
   b. 6-8 cm and 2-4 kg
   c. 8-9 cm and 3-5 kg
   d. 4-6 cm and 3-4 kg

10. The diet of an adolescent in the United States is most likely to be deficient in which of the following nutrients? (Choose 4)
    a. Vitamin C
    b. Energy
    c. Calcium and vitamin D
    d. Protein
    e. Fluoride
    f. Magnesium
    g. Vitamins B_6 and B_{12}
    h. Vitamins A and E

11. What is the best biochemical parameter to use when assessing the nutritional status of a pediatric patient with cancer receiving chemotherapy?
    a. Albumin
    b. Prealbumin
    c. Hemoglobin and hematocrit
    d. Total lymphocyte count

12. A 6-month-old infant weighs 7 kg and is 62 cm in length. He is at the 90% weight for his length. Following GI surgery he is receiving TPN solution consisting of 15% dextrose and 2.5% TrophAmine at 27.7 mL/hr, with 1.5 mL/hr of 20% Intralipid. Which of the following is correct regarding total fluid intake, calories, amino acids, and lipid intake?
    a. 100 cc/kg, 68 kcal/kg, 2.4 g/kg amino acids, 1.1 g/kg lipids
    b. 95 cc/kg, 68 kcal/kg, 2.5 g/kg amino acids, 1.1 g/kg lipids
    c. 100 cc/kg, 82 kcal/kg, 2.4 g/kg amino acids, 0.55 g/kg lipids
    d. 95 cc/kg, 76 kcal/kg, 2.5 g/kg amino acids, 1.1 g/kg lipids

13. A 10-year-old boy with cystic fibrosis presents to the hospital with a BMI at the 5% for his age. What does this indicate?
    a. His nutritional status is still acceptable.
    b. He is at nutrition risk.
    c. He has nutritional failure.
    d. Other parameters are needed for further assessment.

14. A patient with cholestatic liver disease should receive a minimum of which fatty acid to prevent essential fatty acid deficiency?
    a. 3% of calories from eicosapentaenoic acid (EPA)
    b. 3% of calories from docosahexaenoic acid (DHA)
    c. 3% of calories from linolenic acid
    d. 3% of calories from linoleic acid

15. What is the main reason for growth failure in an infant with congenital heart disease (CHD)?
    a. Early satiety
    b. Malabsorption
    c. Inadequate energy intake
    d. Vomiting

16. Which of the following statements is FALSE about determining a nutrition diagnosis?
    a. Dietitians may document a medical diagnosis if there is not an appropriate nutrition diagnosis to choose from.
    b. A nutrition diagnosis is an issue that can be resolved or improved with nutrition intervention.
    c. The nutrition diagnosis should be written in the PES format (Problem, Etiology, Signs/Symptoms).
    d. There may be more than one nutrition diagnosis for the same patient.

17. What would be the best PES statement for a child with newly diagnosed type 1 diabetes who has been referred for initial nutrition counseling?
    a. Excessive carbohydrate intake related to appropriate food choices as evidenced by new diagnosis of diabetes
    b. Food and nutrition knowledge deficit related to lack of prior exposure to accurate nutrition-related information as evidenced by new medical diagnosis of diabetes requiring carbohydrate counting
    c. Excessive oral intake related to food and nutrition knowledge deficit as evidenced by elevated blood glucose levels
    d. Not ready for lifestyle changes related to altered absorption or metabolism as evidenced by type 1 diabetes

18. A family is angry about the excessive diet restrictions for their child in the management of severe chronic kidney disease stage 4 (CKD). This nutrition problem would best be described as
    a. poor nutrition quality of life.
    b. inability to prepare foods and meals.
    c. harmful beliefs and attitudes about food or nutrition.
    d. undesirable food choices.

19. A former 28-week infant born AGA (birth weight 1.1 kg) is now 6 weeks old and 1.7 kg. She is receiving enteral feedings of 140 mL/kg of 24 kcal/ounce premature formula. Half of her feedings are by mouth and the other half is through an NG tube. She has gained an average of 20 g/day over the past week. She is breathing on her own and does not require supplemental oxygen. The baby has the following PES statement as written by the neonatal dietitian: "Suboptimal growth rate related to lack of appropriate weight gain per day as evidenced by average weight gain of 20 grams per day." What are reasonable calorie and protein goals for this infant?
    a. 100 kcal/kg and 2.2 g/kg protein
    b. 120 kcal/kg and 3 g/kg protein
    c. 130 kcal/kg and 4 g/kg protein
    d. 150 kcal/kg and 4.5 g/kg protein

20. A 32-week preterm infant with a birth weight of 1.5 kg is now on day of life 7. He has been receiving trophic feedings along with parenteral nutrition for 2 days. He is tolerating trophic feedings well, and the neonatologist wants to increase enteral feedings. The nutrition diagnosis statement reads: "Inadequate enteral nutrition infusion related to enteral infusion volume not reached as evidenced by infant receiving trophic feedings only on day of life 7." What is a reasonable plan for advancing enteral nutrition?
    a. Increase enteral feedings to 20 mL/kg and advance by 20-40 mL/kg per day.
    b. Increase to 20 mL/kg and advance by 10 mL/kg per day.
    c. Increase to 30 mL/kg and advance by 20-40 mL/kg per day.
    d. Increase by 20 mL/kg every 12 hours up to total fluid goal.

21. Which of the following is not likely to be a nutrition complication for a patient with chylothorax?
    a. Fat-soluble vitamin deficiency
    b. Hypoproteinemia
    c. Metabolic alkalosis
    d. Hypocalcemia

22. What would be a sign that a 3-year-old child may be experiencing osmotic diarrhea?
    a. Diarrhea continues even when all oral intake is stopped.
    b. Diarrhea occurs during a flare of some type of GI disease, such as celiac disease.
    c. Diarrhea resolves after an enteric infection is treated.
    d. Diarrhea ceases when the dietary cause of the diarrhea is removed from the diet.

23. What type of laboratory data would support a nutrition diagnosis of altered nutrition-related laboratory values for a baby with a urea cycle disorder?
    a. Serum glucose
    b. Serum ammonia
    c. Urinary protein
    d. Free carnitine

24. Which of the following would be the most reasonable intervention for a 7-year-old child with newly diagnosed type 1 diabetes?
    a. Teaching the child and family how to manage blood glucose using the diabetic exchange system
    b. Teaching the child and family how to coordinate carbohydrate intake with peak insulin activity to achieve target blood glucose levels using basic carbohydrate counting
    c. Advising the family to remove all sugary foods from the diet and provide a sample meal plan for the child to follow
    d. Calculating the child's energy needs and educate the child and family on the importance of consuming the targeted number of calories each day using 3 meals and 2-3 snacks per day

25. A 4-month-old infant has poor weight gain. The mother has been mixing her infant's formula in the following manner: 1 can of liquid concentrate plus 2 ½ cups water. She lives in a hot climate. What is the potential consequence of this formula dilution?
    a. Hyponatremia
    b. Hyperkalemia
    c. Hypocalcemia
    d. No consequence likely, given the hot climate

26. Bariatric surgery may be appropriate for an adolescent who (Choose 3 options)
   a. has reached Tanner stage 3 or higher.
   b. has reached 95% of adult height based on skeletal survey.
   c. has been unsuccessful in a formalized weight loss program for at least 1 year.
   d. is able to verbalize that surgery is not a cure for obesity.
   e. is able to be responsible for complying with postoperative lifestyle changes that are necessary for long-term success.
   f. has a BMI of 40 or more.

27. A 15-year-old girl is being treated for anorexia nervosa as an outpatient. She is 102 pounds and 64 inches tall. She has lost 15 pounds since over a period of 4 months. What is a safe calorie level to initiate treatment?
   a. Use indirect calorimetry to determine REE.
   b. Use DRI.
   c. Use 50-75% of DRI.
   d. Use BEE x 1.5.

28. A 4-year-old boy weighing 15 kg requires nasogastric feedings during recovery from pneumonia. He has normal GI function. What would be the most appropriate initial feeding regimen?
   a. Isotonic formula started at full strength at 15 mL per hour
   b. Isotonic formula started at half strength at 30 mL per hour
   c. Semi-elemental formula started at half strength at 15 mL per hour
   d. Fluid restricted formula started at 15 mL/hour

29. A former premature infant born at 28 weeks' gestation is now 10 weeks old. The baby gags and turns her head away when attempting to bottle feed. The baby is likely showing signs of
   a. GERD.
   b. aversion to taste of formula.
   c. not being developmentally ready to start oral feeding.
   d. oral aversion.

30. What is the optimal calcium-to-phosphorus ratio (molar ratio) for an infant receiving TPN to help promote adequate bone mineralization?
   a. 1:1
   b. 1.3:1
   c. 1.7:1
   d. 2:1

31. A decision has been made to initiate enteral feedings in a 9-year-old boy with a 30% total body surface area (TBSA) mostly to the arms and lower extremities. He is 8 hours post-injury. He is not intubated but is not yet able to eat. What type of feeding tube is the best recommendation for the burn team?
    a. Nasogastric
    b. PEG
    c. Nasojejunal tube
    d. Nasoduodenal tube

32. What type of study is often recommended by a speech pathologist to evaluate swallow function?
    a. Video fluoroscopy swallow study
    b. CT scan of the throat
    c. Barium swallow
    d. Blue dye swallow study

33. A 20-kg patient has been ordered for parenteral nutrition solution of 15% dextrose, 2% amino acids, 2% Liposyn at 60 cc/hr with standard electrolytes, and multivitamins. The central line is occluded and the nurse wants to run the solution through a peripheral line. What is the potential complication for running this solution through a peripheral line?
    a. Hyperglycemia
    b. Infection
    c. Phlebitis or sclerosis
    d. Fluid overload

34. In counseling a teen about weight control, what is the appropriate recommendation for physical activity?
    a. 30 minutes per day most days
    b. 30 minutes per day of vigorous activity
    c. 60 minutes per day of at least moderate activity
    d. 60 minutes at least 3 times per week of vigorous activity

35. Which of the following is a FALSE statement about product labeling for patients with food allergies or hypersensitivities?
    a. The allergen can be listed below the ingredient list in a statement such as "Contains peanuts."
    b. Advisory labeling such as "Produced on equipment that also processes peanuts" is mandatory.
    c. It is up to the consumer to contact the company for additional information on allergens such as chicken or pork.
    d. The major allergens that are required by law to be listed on the label are egg, milk, soy, peanuts, tree nuts, wheat, fish, and seafood.

36. The Feingold diet is a diet sometimes used to treat
    a. ADHD.
    b. Down syndrome.
    c. elimination diet for food allergies.
    d. obesity.

37. According to the American Academy of Pediatrics, a 2-year-old child should be limited to how much fruit juice per day?
    a. No limit
    b. 12 ounces
    c. 8 ounces
    d. 4 ounces

38. A child with chronic kidney disease who has an elevated parathyroid hormone level would need which of the following diet restrictions?
    a. Low potassium
    b. Low phosphate
    c. Low calcium
    d. Low sodium

39. A 17-year-old girl with cystic fibrosis has been diagnosed with CF-related diabetes. Her BMI is at the 25th percentile for her age. Her physician is prescribing rapid-acting insulin to cover her meals and snacks. Which of the following would NOT be a realistic goal for this patient?
    a. Preprandial blood glucose of 90-180 mg/dL
    b. Bedtime glucose level of 100-180 mg/dL
    c. Blood glucose level of 200 mg/dL or less 2 hours postprandial
    d. Fasting blood glucose levels less than 130 mg/dL

40. An 11-year-old boy with IBD has been on a regular pediatric diet with 2-3 snacks per day. He also tries to drink nutritional supplements. He is now hospitalized. He continues to lose weight and has not been able to increase his oral intake to the established goal of 90% of calorie and protein needs. What is the next step?
    a. Start peripheral parenteral nutrition.
    b. Consult the surgeon for a PICC line and start parenteral nutrition.
    c. Insert an NG tube and start an elemental formula.
    d. Insert an NG tube and initiate a polymeric formula nocturnally.

41. What could be the potential cause of a pediatric patient receiving TPN who is showing signs of apnea, bradycardia, fever, elevated respiration rate, and pulse?
    a. Venous thrombosis
    b. Catheter occlusion
    c. Early sepsis
    d. Pneumothorax

42. Which of the following would be the most compelling reason to suspect NEC in a premature baby receiving enteral nutrition?
    a. Abdominal distention
    b. Mucus residuals
    c. Residuals of undigested milk that is approximately 1.5 times the hourly infused volume
    d. Blood in the stool

43. A malnourished patient showing signs of the refeeding syndrome may have which of the following symptoms? (Choose 5)
    a. Hyperphosphatemia
    b. Hypophosphatemia
    c. Hyperkalemia
    d. Hypokalemia
    e. Hyperglycemia
    f. Hypoglycemia
    g. Low serum magnesium levels
    h. Elevated serum magnesium levels
    i. Cardiac arrhythmias
    j. Dehydration

44. What is the best way to evaluate bone age in an adolescent girl with delayed puberty and a possible eating disorder?
    a. DEXA scan
    b. Right femur radiograph
    c. Left wrist radiograph
    d. Serum calcium, phosphorus, magnesium, and vitamin D levels

45. A 6-year-old boy has been diagnosed with Graft-versus-Host disease (GVHD) following an allogeneic transplant. He has been receiving full TPN support because his GI tract was severely affected with a large volume of watery diarrhea, GI bleeding, cramping, nausea, and vomiting. After 3 weeks, he has been tolerating low-lactose, low-residue isotonic liquids for the past 3 days. What is the next step in the diet progression?
    a. Low-fat, full liquids
    b. Slow introduction of solid food (minimal lactose, very low fat, low fiber)
    c. Advancement to low-fat, minimal lactose diet
    d. Adding one food to the diet per day starting with low-fiber, low-fat foods the child selects

46. Which of the following statements is most accurate about potential clinical or metabolic complications commonly seen in patients receiving HAART?
    a. Alterations in lipid levels, insulin resistance, decreased bone density, redistribution of body fat
    b. Improvement in overall growth, improved bone density, hyperglycemia, hyperlipidemia
    c. Decreased bone density, cholestatic liver disease, hypoglycemia
    d. Growth failure, GI complications, insulin resistance

47. A 14-year-old boy is receiving Stage 2: Structured Weight Management for the treatment of his obesity. He is 240 pounds and 5'11". His BMI is 33.5 and his BMI for age is above the 99th percentile. Nutrition diagnoses include lack of physical activity and excessive energy intake. The initial intervention was to reduce total caloric intake and increase physical activity. What is a reasonable follow-up plan for this boy?
    a. Weekly visits, continued behavioral counseling, and losing 2 pounds per week
    b. Monthly visits, continued behavioral counseling on healthy food choices, a downward trend in BMI for age, logs on screen time, and physical activity
    c. Visits every 2 weeks with referral to Stage 4: Tertiary Care Intervention if goals are not achieved within 3 months
    d. Visits every 3 months; continued behavioral counseling addressing calorie intake, snacking, and healthy food choices; and weight maintenance while growth spurt is anticipated

48. What would NOT be the best way to deliver standardized care for a pediatric burn patient?
    a. Implement standardized order sets for pediatric burn patients based on age and size of burn.
    b. Institute standard orders for feeding tube placement and initiation of enteral nutrition once condition has stabilized.
    c. Institute a standard order for indirect calorimetry within 24 hours of admission.
    d. Initiate nutrition consult and wait until RD has assessed the patient before nutrition interventions are initiated.

49. The NHANES data from 1999-2006 was analyzed to show that the percentage of children ages 12-19 years that had elevated lipid levels was
    a. 15%.
    b. 20%.
    c. 25%.
    d. 30%.

50. What is the name of the landmark research study from 1983-1993 that changed the way diabetes is treated?
    a. Diabetes Control and Complications Trial (DCCT)
    b. The Effects of Glycemic Control on Type 1 Diabetes
    c. Epidemiology of Diabetes Interventions and Complications (EDIC)
    d. Intensive Diabetes Management and Continuous Glucose Monitoring Trial

Answers and Explanations

1. C: A full medical history is required to accurately initiate nutrition assessment in pediatric patients. As much as 15% of children in this country have been identified as having specialized health care issues. Many of these specialized health care needs put the child at risk for nutrition complications. Growth is one area that may be affected, resulting in either under- or overweight children. Disease states or conditions most associated with being overweight or obese include Prader-Willi syndrome and Down syndrome. Disease states or conditions most associated with being underweight include congenital heart disease, fetal alcohol syndrome, cystic fibrosis, prematurity, bronchopulmonary dysplasia, and autistic disorder. Some conditions are also associated with short stature, including cystic fibrosis, cerebral palsy, prematurity, spina bifida, and fetal alcohol syndrome.

2. B: Body mass index (BMI) is the index used most often to evaluate weight status. It is a fairly reliable measure of the amount of adiposity. It does not directly measure body fat. That can only be achieved with the use of underwater weighing or dual energy x-ray absorptiometry (DXA). To calculate BMI, weight in kilograms is divided by height in meters squared. In children, the BMI value is interpreted as a percentile on the NCHS growth chart. This is a comparison of the child's BMI among other children of the same age and sex. A child with a BMI at the 85th percentile is considered overweight and at the 95th percentile or greater is considered obese. A child between the 5th percentile to less than the 95th percentile is considered to be of normal weight and less than the 5th percentile is underweight. Points to consider when interpreting BMI in children and teens is that the amount of body fat will vary with age and the amount of body fat is different between boys and girls.

3. A: Obtaining information about a child's dietary intake is a very important component of the overall nutrition assessment. A 24-hour recall is commonly done but the data collected may be underreported. The previous 24-hour period may not be representative of the usual intake pattern. A diet history may reflect slightly higher intake than normal and is used to assess the normal or usual food pattern. A 7-day food record tends to be the most accurate because it includes both weekdays and weekends; however, the ability to keep detailed records usually wanes as the number of days continues on. A 3-day food record is a good alternative using one weekend day and two weekdays. Food frequencies are sometimes used to determine food patterns but foods tend to be over reported with this method. Innovative technological methods are being developed using smart phones or other computerized methods to help with accuracy for collecting food intake data.

4. B, C, E, F: An allergy to cow's milk protein can present in the first 4 months of an infant's life. The most commonly seen symptoms are the presence of blood in the stool, diarrhea, vomiting or gagging, and colic. Infants may also develop skin

reactions such as atopic dermatitis, hives, or eczema. Respiratory issues such as asthma may occur. Anaphylaxis is rarely seen with cow's milk protein allergy. This is seen more often with allergic reaction to peanuts or tree nuts. Constipation is not a common symptom. Sometimes lactose intolerance is suspected but it is very rare for an infant to have lactose intolerance. Lactose intolerance is a result of an enzyme issue whereas an allergy to cow's milk is an immunologic response. Infants can develop a cow's milk protein allergy while on a cow's-milk-based formula or breast milk.

5. A, E, F, H: Wheat is a difficult ingredient to remove from the diet. With a suspected wheat allergy, it is important to obtain a detailed diet history as well as food frequency questionnaire to determine usual dietary intake patterns. Wheat is found in many products, including baked goods, snack foods, cereals, pastas, soups, and other types of processed foods. Some foods that are not allowed on a wheat free diet include bulgur, couscous, durum, farina, flour, hydrolyzed wheat proteins, pastas, semolina, and triticale. Any ingredient that contains wheat bran, wheat germ, wheat protein isolate, or wheat berries should be avoided. Foods that do not contain wheat include flours made from arrowroot, barley, buckwheat, oats, potato, rye, quinoa, and rice.

6. D: There are a few situations in which breastfeeding is contraindicated. It is important to screen for these issues for any breastfed baby that has been referred for nutrition assessment. These include active use of illicit or street drugs such as heroin, the use of antiretroviral medications, chemotherapy, and radiation therapy. Active tuberculosis that is untreated and HIV infection are also contraindications. A baby with galactosemia cannot receive breast milk because the infant is not able to metabolize galactose. Mothers who have a history of illicit drug use but are in a supervised methadone program may be able to breastfeed their infant. Mothers are encouraged to refrain from drinking alcohol and from smoking cigarettes while breastfeeding because of complications that may occur with the infant.

7. B: Sulfasalazine is an anti-inflammatory medication commonly used to patients with inflammatory bowel syndrome. The symptoms it helps control include diarrhea, abdominal pain, and rectal bleeding. It is used in patients with ulcerative colitis as well as Crohn disease. It may also be used for the treatment of rheumatoid arthritis. This medication may prevent the absorption of folic acid in the intestines and may interfere with folic acid metabolism. Sulfasalazine should be identified as a potential risk factor in the nutrition screening process. It is important to monitor for folate deficiency and megaloblastic anemia. Patients who receive long-term sulfasalazine may need to receive folic acid supplementation.

8. C: The most important factor in the diagnosis of anorexia nervosa in a teenager is weight status. The patient's actual weight needs to be less than 85% of expected weight. In a pediatric patient, this would mean the patient weighs less than the 85th percentile weight for height. The Hamwi method can be used to calculate expected

weight for height where weight is calculated using 100 pounds for the first 5 feet then adding 5 pounds for every inch over 5 feet. The expected weight for height can also be documented on a growth chart. Those with a BMI less than the 5th percentile are at risk for the development of anorexia. Other diagnostic criteria include having a significant fear of gaining weight, a distorted body image, and a loss of 3 or more consecutive menstrual cycles. Other symptoms that may be apparent during nutrition assessment might be a lowered heart rate (less than 60 beats per minute), hypotension, cyanosis of the extremities, dry skin, and the presence of lanugo hair.

9. B: Growth patterns can be categorized into 4 periods. The first period is infancy (birth to age 2). In this period, very rapid growth occurs. Healthy infants normally regain their birth weight within the first week of life, double their birth weight by 5 months, and triple their birth weight by 1 year. In the time between ages 1 and 2, most children will gain 12 cm in height and 2.5 kg in weight on average. Head circumference is also measured and the head will grow approximately 10-11 cm in the first year. During the preschool period (ages 3-6 years), height will increase by approximately 6-8 cm and weight will increase by approximately 2-4 kg per year. In middle childhood (ages 7-10 years), height will increase by an average of 5-6 cm and weight will increase by an average of 2 kg per year. In adolescence (ages 11 to 18 years), girls will grow an average of 8.5-9 cm and boys 9.5- 10.5 cm per year in height.

10. A, C, F, H: The nutrients that are most likely to be deficient in the diet of an adolescent in the United States are vitamins A, D, C, E, calcium, and magnesium. Deficiencies are more likely to occur in areas where the average income is lower, in families that are homeless or have limited access to food, and in Native Americans, but can occur in other areas as well. Calcium and vitamin D deficiency is especially dangerous for this population because peak bone mass occurs during adolescence. Many families will supplement their child's diet with multivitamins; however, the families that supplement are often the ones that do not need supplementation. Additionally, many multivitamins do not contain calcium, which is an important mineral that should be supplemented in many cases.

11. B: Diagnosing malnutrition in a pediatric patient with cancer can be difficult because many of the nutritional markers traditionally used may not be reliable when the patient is receiving chemotherapy or has had multiple blood transfusions. Hemoglobin and hematocrit is one example of parameters that may not truly reflect nutritional status. Total lymphocyte count will be affected by chemotherapy because bone marrow production is suppressed. Serum albumin can be useful in some cases but is more difficult to interpret because the half-life is 20 days. Prealbumin is more useful because the half-life is only 2 days and may correlate better with changes in nutritional status. Prealbumin is less sensitive to changes in fluid status than serum albumin. Both albumin and prealbumin are directly affected by fever and infection but prealbumin is the best laboratory value to use even with its constraints.

12. A: Based on a weight of 7 kg, the TPN solution would provide 27.7 mL/hour + 1.5 mL/hour = 29.2 mL/hour or 700.8 cc per day, to provide 100 mL/kg. The total dextrose intake would be 27.7 mL/hour * 24 hours = 664.8 total mL * 0.15= 99.7 grams of dextrose. There are 3.4 kcal/gram of dextrose or 339 kcal. TrophAmine at 2.5% in 664.8 cc total volume would provide 16.6 grams of amino acids or 2.4 g/kg. There are 4 kcal/gram of amino acids so this would provide 66.5 kcals. At 1.5 mL/hour of Intralipid, there would be a total volume of 36 mL. There are 0.2 g/mL of fat in 20% Intralipid and this would provide 7.2 g of lipids or 1.1 g/kg. There are 10 kcal/g of Intralipid to provide 72 kcal. To convert this to per-kilogram units, total calories would be 339 kcal from dextrose + 66.5 from amino acids + 72 from lipids= 477.5/7 kg= 68 kcal/kg.

13. C: Nutrition is an essential component in the care of patients with cystic fibrosis (CF). A patient with CF should receive a full assessment by a registered dietitian every year at the minimum. Some patients may need to be seen more frequently. Regular anthropometric measurements are essential. Weight and length or height should be measured every 3 months and plotted on the CDC growth charts. Head circumference should also be measured for patients under the age of 2 years. The body mass index percentile is the best way to assess weight and height. Other anthropometric measurements, such as mid-arm muscle circumference and triceps skinfold thickness should be done annually. A patient with CF who is between 2 and 20 years of age who has a BMI/age greater than the 25th percentile is in an acceptable nutritional status. A BMI/age between the 10-25th percentile indicates nutritional risk and a BMI/age less than the 10th percentile is considered to be in nutritional failure. Immediate and aggressive nutrition intervention should begin.

14. D: Essential fatty acids are necessary for normal growth and development. The body can synthesize many of the fatty acids needed, but linoleic and linolenic acid cannot be synthesized. These 2 fatty acids must be ingested in the form of plant-based products such as corn oil or nuts. A patient that has cholestatic liver disease has a reduction in the amount of bile acids produced by the liver and, in turn, long-chain triglycerides (LCT) are not able to be absorbed. With less bile acids available, the body absorbs medium-chain triglycerides (MCT) better because bile is not needed. MCT enters directly into portal circulation. Because LCTs are malabsorbed, essential fatty acid deficiency is likely. At least 3% of calories should be from linoleic acid to help prevent EFA deficiency. Lesser amounts of linolenic acid is required. Linolenic acid is the precursor for EPA and DHA. Patients with cholestatic liver disease are also at risk for fat-soluble vitamin malabsorption because vitamins A, D, E, and K require LCTs to be absorbed.

15. C: The main reason that growth failure occurs in infants with CHD is inadequate caloric intake. It is very difficult for infants to consume enough calories to support growth because the infant has to work so hard to eat, resulting in increased energy expenditure and fatigue. Many times infants with CHD experience tachypnea or rapid breathing. Additionally, decreased cardiac output may cause delayed gastric

emptying. Some infants also experience early satiety or have side effects from the medications they are taking to help their condition. It is important to assess feeding habits of the infant, total intake of formula, and formula preparation methods when initiating nutrition assessment. Social aspects should also be assessed, such as financial ability to provide adequate nutrition and parental efforts at feeding the infant. Growth history needs to be carefully documented and plotted on the appropriate CDC growth charts.

16. A: Step 2 of the Nutrition Care Process is the nutrition diagnosis. This purpose of this step is to identify an issue that can be improved or resolved with appropriate nutrition intervention. A nutrition diagnosis is not a medical diagnosis and the dietitian should not document a medical diagnosis. A comprehensive list is available from the International Dietetics and Nutrition Terminology Reference Manual that contains nutrition diagnosis terms and definitions. If the appropriate term is not found, the nutrition professional should follow the appropriate steps to make an addition to the list. The appropriate format for documenting the nutrition diagnosis is the PES format (Problem, Etiology, Signs/Symptoms). Multiple nutrition diagnoses can be documented for the same patient but PES statements should be limited to issues that are currently being addressed through nutrition intervention. The information obtained during the nutrition assessment step should support the nutrition diagnosis that has been documented.

17. B: A new diagnosis of type 1 diabetes in a child will bring lots of changes and adjustments to the family. Upon initial nutrition consultation, a comprehensive assessment should be completed, including information regarding anthropometrics and growth history; biochemical data such as glucose levels, hemoglobin A_1C, and lipid profile; and social information such as who lives with the child, where the family is currently at emotionally regarding the diagnosis. Information on shopping and cooking practices, prior diabetes knowledge, other family members with diabetes, and any pertinent cultural or religious restrictions should be obtained. The child's normal eating habits, prior special diet, and food frequency is also useful information. Information about school and weekends is also necessary. The most appropriate nutrition PES statement would be related to managing diabetes through nutrition intervention such as carbohydrate counting. The other statement may imply the child did something to cause diabetes or is assumed to be nonadherent prior to nutrition and diabetes education.

18. A: There are 5 stages of chronic kidney disease (CKD). The National Kidney Foundation defines the stage as: Stages 1 and 2 are mild CKD, stage 3 is moderate CKD, stage 4 is severe, and stage 5 is end-stage. Once a child reaches stage 5 CKD, the options are dialysis or transplantation. In stage 4 CKD, the glomerular filtration rate is between 15-29 mL/min/1.73 m^2. This is the immediate pre-dialysis phase. Part of treatment here is diet therapy. Protein is restricted to decrease the amount of urea produced. Sodium and potassium are also restricted, as well as fluid in most cases. An increase in calories is usually required as well to prevent the breakdown

of muscle. Dietary phosphorus is also restricted to prevent the buildup of phosphate in the blood. Many children must take nutritional supplements to help maintain adequate nutrition. It is understandable why the family may be angry about diet restrictions that they have no control over and this affects the overall quality of the child's life.

19. C: A normal rate of weight gain for a preterm infant born at 28 weeks' gestation is approximately 15-35 g/kg. This baby has gained 600 g since birth and is now 34 weeks corrected. Her growth on the Babson growth chart shows a decline in weight from the 50th percentile to just below the 10th percentile. Average weight gain over the past week is approximately 12 g/kg, which is suboptimal. She should be gaining a minimum of 25 g per day with at least 40 g/day desired. She is currently receiving 140 cc/kg of a 24 kcal/oz premature formula. This provides approximately 112 kcal/kg and 3.3 g/kg. A reasonable goal for this infant would be to increase calorie and protein intake to the upper end of the recommended range or 130 kcal/kg and 4 g/kg protein. There are a number of ways to accomplish this, including an increase in total fluid intake, increasing caloric density of formula, and/or changing to a higher protein premature formulation.

20. A: Preterm infants are at risk for many complications including aspiration, necrotizing enterocolitis, and failure to tolerate enteral nutrition. Enteral feedings are always introduced very slowly and advanced carefully to help prevent the development of these complications. Trophic feedings are defined as small-volume feedings generally used for gut stimulation. The volume is usually approximately 10 mL/kg. Trophic feedings are typically given to infants weighing less than 1250 g. This infant is behind on his enteral nutrition. Assuming normal GI function, the feedings could be increased to 20 mL/kg. Advancement can occur at 20-40 kcal/kg per day. Human milk is preferred but premature infant formula should be substituted if breast milk is not available. Human milk fortifier can be added at 4 packets per 100 mL of breast milk when total fluid intake reaches 100 mL/kg.

21. C: A chylothorax can occur as a result of complications from cardiac or thoracic surgery. It may also occur in children with various types of syndromes that involve congenital heart disease such as Down syndrome. The presence of chyle in the pleural space is usually indicative of a chylothorax and can be definitively diagnosed by testing the fluid from the pleural space for white blood cells, triglycerides, and lymphocytes. Chyle is needed for the absorption of long-chain fats and fat-soluble vitamins. Chyle also contains protein and various electrolytes such as sodium and calcium. Large losses of chyle will put a patient at risk for fat-soluble vitamin deficiency and hypoproteinemia. It will also cause hypovolemia, hyponatremia, and hypocalcemia. The pH of chyle fluid is greater than 7 and may cause a metabolic acidosis to occur with loss of chyle.

22. D: Osmotic diarrhea is associated with intolerance to a specific dietary component such as lactose or fructose. The ingestion of sorbitol in elixir-type

medications can also cause osmotic diarrhea. It can also occur with overconsumption of apple juice in toddlers. Diarrhea will stop when the specific item is removed from a child's diet. Secretory diarrhea will not stop even if all oral intake is stopped. It is usually a result of an infection or other condition. A large amount of water is lost with secretory diarrhea. Inflammatory or exudative diarrhea is a result of inflammation from a GI disorder such as celiac disease or Crohn disease. Blood and pus will be found in the stool. Diarrhea can also be due to dysmotility, such as irritable bowel syndrome. It is important to look at the signs and symptoms when trying to make a nutrition diagnosis.

23. B: The American College of Medical Genetics recommends a comprehensive panel of 24 inherited diseases as part of newborn screening. Diseases that can be tested for include amino acid disorders, fatty acid oxidative disorders, organic acid disorders, and many others. Each state has its own screening program in place. Some inborn errors of metabolism are diagnosed at a later age. Early diagnosis is crucial in optimizing outcomes. A urea cycle disorder is an inherited condition that involves nitrogen metabolism such as citrullinemia or argininosuccinic aciduria. Serum ammonia level is an important indicator of a urea cycle disorder. Early intervention is imperative to ameliorate the negative effects of an elevated ammonia level on brain function. Specialized knowledge of inborn errors of metabolism is required to properly care for children with these types of diseases.

24. B: The most appropriate standard of care for a child with newly diagnosed type 1 diabetes is carbohydrate counting. Initially basic carbohydrate counting is taught and advanced carbohydrate counting is gradually incorporated as diabetes management skills increase. The goal for nutrition intervention is to teach the family unit how to coordinate carbohydrate intake with peak insulin activity. The rule of thumb is for every 10-15 g of carbohydrate, 1 unit of rapid-acting insulin is required. Achieving targeted blood glucose levels is the end result. The child and family should be reassured that the child will not have to follow a "diet" and that most of the child's usual foods can be incorporated into their meal plan. Overall healthy eating is the goal not only for the child but for the whole family.

25. A: Proper mixing techniques for infant formula are extremely important. Infant formula comes in 3 forms: powder, liquid concentrate, and ready-to-feed. Standard dilution for liquid concentrate is one 13-oz can plus 13 oz of water to make 20 calories per oz. The recipe the mother has been using provides approximately 15.8 calories per oz. This can be extremely dangerous especially for an infant to under dilute infant formula. There is a risk for hyponatremia, water intoxication, and dilution of the nutrients. This should never be done without physician supervision, even in hot climates. Some parents may underdilute formula to save money and most parents do not know it is dangerous. Standard dilution for powdered formula is one scoop to 2 oz of water. Ready-to-feed infant formula should never be diluted. The appropriate method for mixing infant formula should be reviewed with the mother to prevent complications and achieve normal weight gain.

26. B, D, E: Adolescents are now being considered for bariatric surgery; however, strict criteria have been established for eligibility. Adolescents must be close to fully grown, which includes a Tanner stage of 4 and 95% of adult height achieved based on complete skeletal examination. The body mass index (BMI) must be at least 50 without comorbidities. If testing has identified certain comorbidities, such as elevated fasting glucose, abnormal lipid or liver profiles, or low vitamin B_1, B_{12} and folate levels, the BMI can be 40 or more. At least 6 months of a formal weight loss program must be attempted before bariatric surgery can be considered. The adolescent must be mentally mature enough to understand that bariatric surgery is not a cure for obesity, be able to understand the risks involved with bariatric surgery, and be able to implement the lifestyle changes necessary for long-term success. It is important to understand that the research in this area is still incomplete regarding the safety and long-term results of this surgery on adolescents.

27. C: In outpatient treatment of anorexia nervosa, the goals are to improve eating habits and behaviors, achieve a healthy weight, and address psychological and behavioral issues related to disordered eating. This must be done in a sensitive manner because patients with eating disorders are often very afraid of weight gain and changing eating behaviors. A meal plan needs to be developed that takes into account safe foods as well as additional nutrient-dense foods incorporated into 3 meals and 1-2 snacks per day. Initial energy requirements for outpatient therapy should be approximately 50-75% of the dietary reference intake (in this case approximately 1200-1800 calories). This may not be immediately achievable but should be the goal. Calories will then need to be adjusted to achieve a 0.5-1 lb/week weight gain. Sometimes patients with anorexia will require up to twice the DRI to achieve weight gain. Protein should comprise 15-20% of total calories, 50-60% as carbohydrate and 20-25% as fat.

28. A: There are many different ways to initiate enteral feedings in infants, children, and adolescents. Decisions are usually based on age, status of GI function, current medical issues, nutritional status, and nutrient requirements. Typically isotonic formulations are the first choice. Isotonic formulas do not need to be diluted unless there is a particular concern regarding GI function. Diluting formulas increases the risk of bacterial contamination. It is generally safe to initiate the rate of enteral feedings through a nasogastric tube at 1-2 mL/kg/hr for children weighing less than 35 kg and at 1 mL/kg/hr for children weighing more than 35 kg. The rate may be advanced gradually up to the goal rate within 24-48 hours. The rate and strength (if diluted) should not be advanced at the same time. Careful monitoring is required as tube feedings advance. If intolerance occurs, the regimen should be returned to the previously tolerated rate.

29. D: Premature babies are at risk for developing oral aversion because they have been exposed to intubation, prolonged placement of either nasogastric or orogastric

tubes for feeding and frequent suctioning. All of this signifies negative sensory stimuli to the oral area. When it is time to begin working on oral feedings, many premature babies do not show interest, cry, turn their head away, or gag or wretch when bottle feeding or breast feeding is introduced. These infants often do not possess normal hunger cues either because they have been fed with tube feedings. Early positive and pleasant stimuli to the face should be introduced, such as offering a pacifier when the tube feeding is being delivered or to help soothe the baby. Oral feedings should be started as soon as medically possible and not delayed unnecessarily. Enlisting the help of a pediatric speech pathologist or occupational therapist will help with the transition.

30. B: Newborns and infants have higher calcium requirements related to bone mineralization. The optimal calcium: phosphorus molar ratio is 1.3:1. By weight, it is 1.7:1. It is often difficult to meet the calcium and phosphorus requirements for high-risk infants, especially if the infant is fluid-restricted. There is a chance that high concentrations of these 2 mineral will cause a precipitate to occur, which may cause phlebitis or emboli. There are other factors that affect how much calcium and phosphorus can be safely added to a solution, such as low amino acid content, low dextrose concentration, and a high pH level. The addition of L-cysteine to neonatal TPN solutions help improve the pH level. L-cysteine is added at 40 mg/g of amino acid. It is important to confer with the pediatric pharmacist or nutrition support pharmacist regarding safe levels of calcium and phosphorus in a solution.

31. D: Nutrition support to a patient with a burn injury should begin as soon as medically possible. Significant deficits can develop if enteral nutrition is delayed. Aggressive nutrition has been demonstrated to improve tolerance to tube feedings and helps to maintain the integrity of the bowel, preventing bacterial translocation. Early initiation of enteral nutrition will also help to blunt the hypermetabolic response to injury and help to maintain nitrogen balance. Tube feedings into the stomach are not recommended initially after a burn injury because a gastric ileus is often present. The ileus will prevent the tube feeding from being tolerated and advanced to full volume and calorie goals. Gastric feedings also increase the risk for aspiration during dressing changes, physical therapy and surgery. A feeding tube paced into the lower third part of the duodenum is the best option. It is safer for the patient, even during surgery, dressing changes, or during emergency treatment such as resuscitation.

32. A: A video fluoroscopy swallow study (VFSS) is also known as an esophagram or modified barium swallow. It is a test used to determine if food is being swallowed appropriately and not being aspirated into the airway. The test also determines if there are any areas of the mouth and throat that are not functioning appropriately. The test can help the speech language pathologist (SLP) determine the safest foods the patient should be able to swallow, as well as strategies for improving swallow function such as positioning. The SLP will work closely with the medical team and dietitian to determine the appropriate consistency and what type of thickeners to

use, if any. The dietitian will make sure nutrient and fluid needs will be appropriately met and ensure the length of time needed for supplemental tube feedings. The use of blue dye is no longer recommended due to the risk for infection and other complications.

33. C: It is extremely important to be aware of the type of solution being administered and the type of venous catheter available. The solution as ordered most likely has been labeled as a central solution, which must be recognized and administered appropriately. A peripheral line should have a maximum osmolarity of 900 mOsm/L. This is typically a restriction in both dextrose concentration of 10% and 2% amino acid concentration with added electrolytes. 15% dextrose has an osmolarity of approximately 750 mOsm/L and the osmolarity of the amino acids are approximately 280 mOsm/L. Just the dextrose and amino acids contribute 1030 mOsm/L, which exceeds the safe limit. Administering a very concentrated solution through a peripheral line would increase the risk of developing phlebitis or sclerosis or cause tissue sloughing, similar to a chemical burn. The safest alternative would be to run an IV solution appropriate for a peripheral line until central access is reestablished.

34. C: Physical activity is an important component in addressing weight control. In addition to burning calories, physical activity helps reduce the risk of heart disease, diabetes, cancer, and other diseases. It also provides mental benefits, such as reducing depression and improving overall attitude. At least 60 min/day of moderate activity is recommended, and one hour of vigorous activity at least 3 times per week is advised. The more time that is spent being inactive, such as watching TV, playing video games, or using the computer increases the risk of obesity. There are many barriers to children and adolescents meeting physical activity goals. Safety is often cited as an issue, especially for children who live in higher crime areas, have more traffic, or lack access to community or recreation programs. Physical activity is important, however, and works collaboratively with diet in trying to control weight issues.

35. B: In 2006, a newly revised labeling law went into effect called the Food Allergen Labeling and Consumer Protection Act. This law requires that the 8 main allergens (egg, milk, soy, peanuts, tree nuts, wheat, fish, and seafood) are plainly identified on the label of any packaged food. It is up to the consumer to contact the manufacturer for the presence of other allergens, such as chicken, pork, or a specific tree nut. The potential allergen can be identified in 3 ways. The first is inclusion on the ingredient list. The second way is clarification of a technical or scientific term in parentheses such as lactalbumin (e.g., milk). The third way is under the ingredient list a statement can be made such as "Contains milk." Advisory labeling is a statement made on the label such as "processed in a facility that also processes peanuts" or "may be processed on equipment that also processes peanuts." This is voluntary. Consumers must contact the manufacturer for information regarding cross-contamination, especially for highly allergic individuals.

36. A: The Feingold diet is a diet popular in the 1970s in the treatment of attention deficit hyperactivity disorder (ADHD). The diet removed artificial flavorings, colorings, and additives from the diet with the assumption that behavior would improve. There has not been substantial scientific data to support this diet; however, anecdotally families have found some relief of behavioral problems with the implementation of this diet. The diet eliminates all processed foods containing preservatives, coloring, and natural salicylates such as fruits. A modified version of the diet that does include fruit can be helpful to children and can be nutritionally sound with proper counseling by a registered dietitian.

37. D: Fruit juice can be a problematic beverage for children. It may replace other fluids, such as milk and water. Too much fruit juice in a toddler's diet can cause diarrhea, may replace food in the diet, and may contribute to excessive weight gain. The American Academy of Pediatrics (AAP) recommends that children between the ages of 1 and 6 be limited to 4-6 oz of fruit juice each day. Children older than 7 may have 8-12 oz of fruit juice per day. The AAP suggests that a child may actually have higher intakes of minerals and vitamins if half of the fruit servings were from 100% fruit juice as long as the other half of the fruit servings were from whole fruit. The use of sweetened beverages, such as soda or fruit punch, should be restricted due to the risk for obesity. It is also important for young children to include milk and milk products. Four ½-cup servings of milk (or milk substitutes) are recommended for 2-3-year-old children.

38. B: Children with chronic kidney disease have difficulty removing excess phosphorus from their blood. Hyperphosphatemia can lead to hypocalcemia, which in turn can lead to bone disease. Vitamin D also plays a role in phosphorus metabolism because vitamin D is converted to 1,25 dihydroxycholecalciferol in the kidneys. When the kidneys aren't working properly, a deficiency can develop which can lead to secondary hyperparathyroidism. Typically phosphorus will need to be restricted to 800-1000 mg/day. Phosphorus is found in foods such as milk, cheese, yogurt, pudding, meats, nuts, seeds, and soda. Phosphorus is not required to be listed on the nutrient label so it is important to educate the family about sources of phosphorus. Many patients will also require phosphorus binders to help reduce the amount of phosphorus by binding with phosphorus in the intestines. A vitamin D supplement in the form of calcitriol is also required.

39. C: Children with cystic fibrosis are living longer with improvement in the treatment of this disease. Many individuals who have CF are now being diagnosed with CF-related diabetes (CFRD). This occurs in at least 13% of patients and is usually diagnosed between the ages of 18 and 21. Management of CFRD is similar to diabetes mellitus; however, there are some distinct differences. Because of the risk for malnutrition, calorie restriction is never indicated. A high-calorie and high-fat diet remain the recommendation, with 40% of total calories from fat and 20% from protein. Patients with CFRD do have the risk for developing microvascular

complications, so it is imperative to maintain good glucose levels. Fasting blood glucose levels should be less than 130 mg/dL, preprandial glucose levels should be 90-180 mg/dL, and postprandial levels should be less than 180 mg/dL. Glucose levels at bedtime should be between 100 mg/dL and 180 mg/dL. The glucose level will dictate the amount of carbohydrate required at a meal or snack.

40. D: The nutritional status of patients with inflammatory bowel disease is often compromised. Calorie requirements can be calculated in many different ways, ranging from the Estimated Energy Requirements (EER) to basal metabolic rate increased by a stress factor of 1.3-1.5. Some patients will also need catch-up growth calculated. Protein needs are usually elevated at 1.5-2 g/kg. If this patient is unable to meet the established goal of 90% of requirements, the next step would be to place a feeding tube. A nasogastric or nasoenteric tube is appropriate initially, but a more permanent tube may need to be considered if oral intake does not improve. A polymeric formula has been shown to be as successful as elemental formulas. Patients over the age of 13 may be considered for an adult formula rather than a pediatric formulation. The feeding schedule should be determined based on oral intake. Often a bolus schedule during the day or a continuous nocturnal tube feeding are helpful in maintaining the quality of life for children.

41. C: Patient monitoring during parenteral nutrition is extremely important. Changes in vital signs, including temperature, respiration rate, pulse, and blood pressure can be an early indication that sepsis or some other complication may be developing. Laboratory monitoring is also essential, as sudden hyperglycemia or an elevated white blood cell count may also indicate infection. A child that exhibits any signs of sepsis should be treated immediately. Bacterial, fungal, or other types of infections can occur at the hub or at the skin entrance site. Proper catheter care can help to minimize infectious complications, including dressing changes every 48-72 hours or per hospital policy, and changing the catheter tubing every 48 hours. Strict aseptic technique is required at all times during catheter care.

42. D: Necrotizing enterocolitis (NEC) is a potentially devastating complication for a premature infant. Continual assessment of feeding tolerance is imperative in order to detect the early stages of NEC and begin treatment. There are no universal guidelines for feeding tolerance. Monitoring of the infant coupled with clinical observations is important. Continued apnea, bradycardia, and temperature instability can be early warning signs. Blood in the stool or in the residuals may be an indication of NEC. Monitoring of residuals can be subjective but in general, undigested milk residuals of 50% of a bolus feeding or 1.5 times an hourly infusion rate are considered acceptable in the absence of other symptoms. Mucus residuals may occur immediately after a lung infection. Bile in the residuals may indicate tube migration or something more serious. Abdominal distention may be a result of swallowed air or insufficient bowel movements. Visible loops of bowel seen on x-ray may indicate NEC or other illness.

43. B, D, E, G, I: Refeeding syndrome can occur when initiating aggressive nutrition support in a patient with malnutrition. Essentially the body goes into a shock state when excessive calories are provided, causing an increase in insulin release. The increase in insulin release causes an alteration in glucose metabolism because of the increased uptake of glucose at the cellular level. Hypophosphatemia is the hallmark of the refeeding syndrome, which can lead to changes in both cardiac and respiratory function. Other metabolic changes that can occur include hypokalemia, which can also cause cardiac disturbances, and low serum magnesium levels, which can contribute to cardiac arrhythmias and changes in GI function. As the shift of electrolytes into the intracellular space and the shift of glucose into the cells for oxidation occur, there is a decrease in sodium and fluid excretion, causing the potential for fluid imbalance in the body putting an additional strain on the body.

44. C: A left wrist radiograph including the hand and fingers is the best way to measure the degree of maturity of the skeletal system. It is a safe procedure and does not inflict any pain on a child. This x-ray will look at the growth plate, which is easy to identify on x-ray because they are softer due to less mineral content and they appear darker than regular bone on x-ray. The x-ray can determine when the child will enter puberty, how chronological age and bone age compare, what the end height will be, and how much time is left in the growth process. Anorexia nervosa can delay both puberty and bone development. Low body weight can cause the body to stop producing estrogen, which in turn will impact bone density. Eating disorders may also prevent the attainment of peak bone mass. Individuals with anorexia will most likely have a bone age that is lower than their actual chronological age.

45. B: Graft-versus-Host disease (GVHD) can develop in patients who have had an allogenic transplant. It is an immunologic response in which the new stem cells that have been received attack the host's tissue antigens. Severe organ damage can result and may affect the skin, GI tract, or liver. Common symptoms are nausea, vomiting, severe watery diarrhea, GI bleeding, and abdominal cramping. Often TPN is required until symptoms begin to subside. There are 5 stages in the nutritional treatment. The first is bowel rest with TPN. The second is slow introduction of oral diet using low lactose and isotonic low-residue liquids. The third step is very slow introduction of solids every 3-4 hours using minimal lactose, very low fat, and low fiber, with no gastric irritants or acidic foods. The next 2 steps are designed to work toward progression to a regular diet based on overall tolerance to the diet. This would include monitoring for cramping, bowel movements, and serum albumin levels. TPN would continue until a full diet is achieved.

46. A: Highly active antiretroviral therapy (HAART) is the gold standard for treating patients with HIV infection. There over 17 drugs available for use in the pediatric population. There are 6 main categories for HAART and each category works on specific areas. The categories are nucleoside/nucleotide reverse transcriptase inhibitors (NRTIs/NtRTIs), non-nucleoside analogue reverse transcriptase inhibitors (NNRTIs), protease inhibitors (PIs), entry inhibitors, and integrase

inhibitors. Most often these drugs are used in specific combinations. The goal of therapy is to reduce the patient's viral load and promote the CD4 count to rise. With the use of HAART, life expectancy is growing. Some of the clinical and metabolic complications of this therapy are redistribution of body fat called lipodystrophy, insulin resistance, decreased bone density, and abnormal lipid levels. Nutrition intervention is very important in addressing these issues and preventing malnutrition. Ongoing education is required for caregivers regarding appropriate food choices, food safety, optimal growth, and dietary modifications.

47. B: In Stage 2: Structured Weight Management, the initial plan is typically the development of a structured meal plan for meals and snacks, healthy food choices, and an overall balanced diet. Physical activity should be addressed with a goal of reducing the amount of screen time (TV, computer, etc.) to less than 1-2 hours per day and increasing the amount of time spent engaging in physical activity. Asking the boy to keep a detailed log of activities is helpful in evaluating success. In terms of weight loss, the best goal would be for a continued downward trend in BMI for age to eventually reach below the 85th percentile. Some children may require a slow, gradual weight loss, while others will require weight maintenance while height increases. Monthly follow-ups at this point are realistic. After 3-6 months of counseling and monitoring, reassessment is needed to determine if sufficient progress is being made or if the patient needs additional support or referral to stage 4.

48. D: Protocols or standardized order sets are a good way to initiate nutrition interventions for certain disease states or conditions such as burn injury. Pediatric patients with a burn injury will require certain pieces of information to get the assessment started, including indirect calorimetry, certain laboratory data such as serum prealbumin, or 24-hour urinary urea collection to determine nitrogen balance. The medical team does not need to wait for the registered dietitian to ask for this information; it can be done automatically. Additionally, the standard of care for burn injury is to start enteral nutrition as soon as medically feasible; therefore, a standard order for placing a feeding tube into the appropriate location and starting tube feedings with a preselected formula is acceptable. Consultation with the registered dietitian is needed; however, nutrition interventions do not need to wait until the patient has been fully assessed by the RD.

49. B: Data that was analyzed from the National Health and Nutrition Examination Survey (NHANES) from 1999-2006 showed that approximately 20% of children between 12 and 19 years of age had elevated lipid levels. This is extremely alarming given the sharp increase in obesity rates. The National Cholesterol Education Program (NCEP) and the American Heart Association (AHA) have collaborated to develop the Therapeutic Lifestyle Changes (TLC) diet and promotes this healthy diet for children over the age of 2. This is particularly important for children with a family history of heart disease. The diet consists of 50-60% of total calories from carbohydrate, 15% from protein, and 25-25% of total calories from fat. Less than

7% of calories from saturated fat is recommended. The addition of plant stanols and sterols is advocated as well as increasing the amount of soluble fiber. Fat restriction is not recommended for children under the age of 2 due to the developing brain.

50. A: The Diabetes Control and Complications Trial (DCCT) was conducted from 1983-1993. This trial provided groundbreaking data that changed the way diabetes is treated. The study looked at the effects of standard diabetes care compared with intensive control on the development of complications. The trial showed that keeping the hemoglobin A1C level at 6% or less significantly reduced complications such as retinopathy, kidney disease, neuropathy, and cardiovascular disease. The trial enabled evidence-based care models to be developed to help standardize the treatment of diabetes. The DCCT also demonstrated that a team approach to treating diabetes is extremely important in achieving management goals. Pediatric endocrine clinics are often based on information obtained from this trial, such as involving a pediatric child life specialist to help the child navigate an appointment.

Secret Key #1 - Time is Your Greatest Enemy

Pace Yourself

Wear a watch. At the beginning of the test, check the time (or start a chronometer on your watch to count the minutes), and check the time after every few questions to make sure you are "on schedule."

If you are forced to speed up, do it efficiently. Usually one or more answer choices can be eliminated without too much difficulty. Above all, don't panic. Don't speed up and just begin guessing at random choices. By pacing yourself, and continually monitoring your progress against your watch, you will always know exactly how far ahead or behind you are with your available time. If you find that you are one minute behind on the test, don't skip one question without spending any time on it, just to catch back up. Take 15 fewer seconds on the next four questions, and after four questions you'll have caught back up. Once you catch back up, you can continue working each problem at your normal pace.

Furthermore, don't dwell on the problems that you were rushed on. If a problem was taking up too much time and you made a hurried guess, it must be difficult. The difficult questions are the ones you are most likely to miss anyway, so it isn't a big loss. It is better to end with more time than you need than to run out of time.

Lastly, sometimes it is beneficial to slow down if you are constantly getting ahead of time. You are always more likely to catch a careless mistake by working more slowly than quickly, and among very high-scoring test takers (those who are likely to have lots of time left over), careless errors affect the score more than mastery of material.

Secret Key #2 - Guessing is not Guesswork

You probably know that guessing is a good idea - unlike other standardized tests, there is no penalty for getting a wrong answer. Even if you have no idea about a question, you still have a 20-25% chance of getting it right.

Most test takers do not understand the impact that proper guessing can have on their score. Unless you score extremely high, guessing will significantly contribute to your final score.

Monkeys Take the Test

What most test takers don't realize is that to insure that 20-25% chance, you have to guess randomly. If you put 20 monkeys in a room to take this test, assuming they answered once per question and behaved themselves, on average they would get 20-25% of the questions correct. Put 20 test takers in the room, and the average will be much lower among guessed questions. Why?

1. The test writers intentionally writes deceptive answer choices that "look" right. A test taker has no idea about a question, so picks the "best looking" answer, which is often wrong. The monkey has no idea what looks good and what doesn't, so will consistently be lucky about 20-25% of the time.

2. Test takers will eliminate answer choices from the guessing pool based on a hunch or intuition. Simple but correct answers often get excluded, leaving a 0% chance of being correct. The monkey has no clue, and often gets lucky with the best choice.

This is why the process of elimination endorsed by most test courses is flawed and detrimental to your performance- test takers don't guess, they make an ignorant stab in the dark that is usually worse than random.

$5 Challenge

Let me introduce one of the most valuable ideas of this course- the $5 challenge:

You only mark your "best guess" if you are willing to bet $5 on it.

You only eliminate choices from guessing if you are willing to bet $5 on it.

Why $5? Five dollars is an amount of money that is small yet not insignificant, and can really add up fast (20 questions could cost you $100). Likewise, each answer choice on one question of the test will have a small impact on your overall score, but it can really add up to a lot of points in the end.

The process of elimination IS valuable. The following shows your chance of guessing it right:

If you eliminate wrong answer choices until only this many remain:	1	2	3
Chance of getting it correct:	100%	50%	33%

However, if you accidentally eliminate the right answer or go on a hunch for an incorrect answer, your chances drop dramatically: to 0%. By guessing among all the answer choices, you are GUARANTEED to have a shot at the right answer.

That's why the $5 test is so valuable- if you give up the advantage and safety of a pure guess, it had better be worth the risk.

What we still haven't covered is how to be sure that whatever guess you make is truly random. Here's the easiest way:

Always pick the first answer choice among those remaining.

Such a technique means that you have decided, **before you see a single test question**, exactly how you are going to guess- and since the order of choices tells you nothing about which one is correct, this guessing technique is perfectly random.

This section is not meant to scare you away from making educated guesses or eliminating choices- you just need to define when a choice is worth eliminating. The $5 test, along with a pre-defined random guessing strategy, is the best way to make sure you reap all of the benefits of guessing.

Secret Key #3 - Practice Smarter, Not Harder

Many test takers delay the test preparation process because they dread the awful amounts of practice time they think necessary to succeed on the test. We have refined an effective method that will take you only a fraction of the time.

There are a number of "obstacles" in your way to succeed. Among these are answering questions, finishing in time, and mastering test-taking strategies. All must be executed on the day of the test at peak performance, or your score will suffer. The test is a mental marathon that has a large impact on your future.

Just like a marathon runner, it is important to work your way up to the full challenge. So first you just worry about questions, and then time, and finally strategy:

Success Strategy

1. Find a good source for practice tests.
2. If you are willing to make a larger time investment, consider using more than one study guide- often the different approaches of multiple authors will help you "get" difficult concepts.
3. Take a practice test with no time constraints, with all study helps "open book." Take your time with questions and focus on applying strategies.
4. Take a practice test with time constraints, with all guides "open book."
5. Take a final practice test with no open material and time limits

If you have time to take more practice tests, just repeat step 5. By gradually exposing yourself to the full rigors of the test environment, you will condition your mind to the stress of test day and maximize your success.

Secret Key #4 - Prepare, Don't Procrastinate

Let me state an obvious fact: if you take the test three times, you will get three different scores. This is due to the way you feel on test day, the level of preparedness you have, and, despite the test writers' claims to the contrary, some tests WILL be easier for you than others.

Since your future depends so much on your score, you should maximize your chances of success. In order to maximize the likelihood of success, you've got to prepare in advance. This means taking practice tests and spending time learning the information and test taking strategies you will need to succeed.

Never take the test as a "practice" test, expecting that you can just take it again if you need to. Feel free to take sample tests on your own, but when you go to take the official test, be prepared, be focused, and do your best the first time!

Secret Key #5 - Test Yourself

Everyone knows that time is money. There is no need to spend too much of your time or too little of your time preparing for the test. You should only spend as much of your precious time preparing as is necessary for you to get the score you need.

Once you have taken a practice test under real conditions of time constraints, then you will know if you are ready for the test or not.

If you have scored extremely high the first time that you take the practice test, then there is not much point in spending countless hours studying. You are already there.

Benchmark your abilities by retaking practice tests and seeing how much you have improved. Once you score high enough to guarantee success, then you are ready.

If you have scored well below where you need, then knuckle down and begin studying in earnest. Check your improvement regularly through the use of practice tests under real conditions. Above all, don't worry, panic, or give up. The key is perseverance!

Then, when you go to take the test, remain confident and remember how well you did on the practice tests. If you can score high enough on a practice test, then you can do the same on the real thing.

General Strategies

The most important thing you can do is to ignore your fears and jump into the test immediately- do not be overwhelmed by any strange-sounding terms. You have to jump into the test like jumping into a pool- all at once is the easiest way.

Make Predictions

As you read and understand the question, try to guess what the answer will be. Remember that several of the answer choices are wrong, and once you begin reading them, your mind will immediately become cluttered with answer choices designed to throw you off. Your mind is typically the most focused immediately after you have read the question and digested its contents. If you can, try to predict what the correct answer will be. You may be surprised at what you can predict.

Quickly scan the choices and see if your prediction is in the listed answer choices. If it is, then you can be quite confident that you have the right answer. It still won't hurt to check the other answer choices, but most of the time, you've got it!

Answer the Question

It may seem obvious to only pick answer choices that answer the question, but the test writers can create some excellent answer choices that are wrong. Don't pick an answer just because it sounds right, or you believe it to be true. It MUST answer the question. Once you've made your selection, always go back and check it against the question and make sure that you didn't misread the question, and the answer choice does answer the question posed.

Benchmark

After you read the first answer choice, decide if you think it sounds correct or not. If it doesn't, move on to the next answer choice. If it does, mentally mark that answer choice. This doesn't mean that you've definitely selected it as your answer choice, it just means that it's the best you've seen thus far. Go ahead and read the next choice. If the next choice is worse than the one you've already selected, keep going to the next answer choice. If the next choice is better than the choice you've already selected, mentally mark the new answer choice as your best guess.

The first answer choice that you select becomes your standard. Every other answer choice must be benchmarked against that standard. That choice is correct until proven otherwise by another answer choice beating it out. Once you've decided that no other answer choice seems as good, do one final check to ensure that your answer choice answers the question posed.

Valid Information

Don't discount any of the information provided in the question. Every piece of information may be necessary to determine the correct answer. None of the information in the question is there to throw you off (while the answer choices will certainly have information to throw you off). If two seemingly unrelated topics are discussed, don't ignore either. You can be confident there is a relationship, or it wouldn't be included in the question, and you are probably going to have to determine what is that relationship to find the answer.

Avoid "Fact Traps"

Don't get distracted by a choice that is factually true. Your search is for the answer that answers the question. Stay focused and don't fall for an answer that is true but incorrect. Always go back to the question and make sure you're choosing an answer that actually answers the question and is not just a true statement. An answer can be factually correct, but it MUST answer the question asked. Additionally, two answers can both be seemingly correct, so be sure to read all of the answer choices, and make sure that you get the one that BEST answers the question.

Milk the Question

Some of the questions may throw you completely off. They might deal with a subject you have not been exposed to, or one that you haven't reviewed in years. While your lack of knowledge about the subject will be a hindrance, the question itself can give you many clues that will help you find the correct answer. Read the question carefully and look for clues. Watch particularly for adjectives and nouns describing difficult terms or words that you don't recognize. Regardless of if you completely understand a word or not, replacing it with a synonym either provided or one you more familiar with may help you to understand what the questions are asking. Rather than wracking your mind about specific detailed information concerning a difficult term or word, try to use mental substitutes that are easier to understand.

The Trap of Familiarity

Don't just choose a word because you recognize it. On difficult questions, you may not recognize a number of words in the answer choices. The test writers don't put "make-believe" words on the test; so don't think that just because you only recognize all the words in one answer choice means that answer choice must be correct. If you only recognize words in one answer choice, then focus on that one. Is it correct? Try your best to determine if it is correct. If it is, that is great, but if it doesn't, eliminate it. Each word and answer choice you eliminate increases your chances of getting the question correct, even if you then have to guess among the unfamiliar choices.

Eliminate Answers

Eliminate choices as soon as you realize they are wrong. But be careful! Make sure you consider all of the possible answer choices. Just because one appears right, doesn't mean that the next one won't be even better! The test writers will usually put more than one good answer choice for every question, so read all of them. Don't worry if you are stuck between two that seem right. By getting down to just two remaining possible choices, your odds are now 50/50. Rather than wasting too much time, play the odds. You are guessing, but guessing wisely, because you've been able to knock out some of the answer choices that you know are wrong. If you are eliminating choices and realize that the last answer choice you are left with is also obviously wrong, don't panic. Start over and consider each choice again. There may easily be something that you missed the first time and will realize on the second pass.

Tough Questions

If you are stumped on a problem or it appears too hard or too difficult, don't waste time. Move on! Remember though, if you can quickly check for obviously incorrect answer choices, your chances of guessing correctly are greatly improved. Before you completely give up, at least try to knock out a couple of possible answers. Eliminate what you can and then guess at the remaining answer choices before moving on.

Brainstorm

If you get stuck on a difficult question, spend a few seconds quickly brainstorming. Run through the complete list of possible answer choices. Look at each choice and ask yourself, "Could this answer the question satisfactorily?" Go through each answer choice and consider it independently of the other. By systematically going through all possibilities, you may find something that you would otherwise overlook. Remember that when you get stuck, it's important to try to keep moving.

Read Carefully

Understand the problem. Read the question and answer choices carefully. Don't miss the question because you misread the terms. You have plenty of time to read each question thoroughly and make sure you understand what is being asked. Yet a happy medium must be attained, so don't waste too much time. You must read carefully, but efficiently.

Face Value

When in doubt, use common sense. Always accept the situation in the problem at face value. Don't read too much into it. These problems will not require you to make huge leaps of logic. The test writers aren't trying to throw you off with a cheap trick. If you have to go beyond creativity and make a leap of logic in order to have an answer choice answer the question, then you should look at the other answer choices. Don't overcomplicate the problem by creating theoretical relationships or explanations that will warp time or space. These are normal problems rooted in reality. It's just that the applicable relationship or explanation may not be readily apparent and you have to figure things out. Use your common sense to interpret anything that isn't clear.

Prefixes

If you're having trouble with a word in the question or answer choices, try dissecting it. Take advantage of every clue that the word might include. Prefixes and suffixes can be a huge help. Usually they allow you to determine a basic meaning. Pre- means before, post- means after, pro - is positive, de- is negative. From these prefixes and suffixes, you can get an idea of the general meaning of the word and try to put it into context. Beware though of any traps. Just because con is the opposite of pro, doesn't necessarily mean congress is the opposite of progress!

Hedge Phrases

Watch out for critical "hedge" phrases, such as likely, may, can, will often, sometimes, often, almost, mostly, usually, generally, rarely, sometimes. Question writers insert these hedge phrases to cover every possibility. Often an answer choice will be wrong simply because it leaves no room for exception. Avoid answer choices that have definitive words like "exactly," and "always".

Switchback Words

Stay alert for "switchbacks". These are the words and phrases frequently used to alert you to shifts in thought. The most common switchback word is "but". Others include although, however, nevertheless, on the other hand, even though, while, in spite of, despite, regardless of.

New Information

Correct answer choices will rarely have completely new information included. Answer choices typically are straightforward reflections of the material asked about and will directly relate to the question. If a new piece of information is included in an answer choice that doesn't even seem to relate to the topic being asked about, then that answer choice is likely incorrect. All of the information needed to answer the question is usually provided for you, and so you should not have to make guesses that are unsupported or choose answer choices that require unknown information that cannot be reasoned on its own.

Time Management

On technical questions, don't get lost on the technical terms. Don't spend too much time on any one question. If you don't know what a term means, then since you don't have a dictionary, odds are you aren't going to get much further. You should immediately recognize terms as whether or not you know them. If you don't, work with the other clues that you have, the other answer choices and terms provided, but don't waste too much time trying to figure out a difficult term.

Contextual Clues

Look for contextual clues. An answer can be right but not correct. The contextual clues will help you find the answer that is most right and is correct. Understand the context in which a phrase or statement is made. This will help you make important distinctions.

Don't Panic

Panicking will not answer any questions for you. Therefore, it isn't helpful. When you first see the question, if your mind goes blank, take a deep breath. Force yourself to mechanically go through the steps of solving the problem and using the strategies you've learned.

Pace Yourself

Don't get clock fever. It's easy to be overwhelmed when you're looking at a page full of questions, your mind is full of random thoughts and feeling confused, and the clock is ticking down faster than you would like. Calm down and maintain the pace that you have set for yourself. As long as you are on track by monitoring your pace, you are guaranteed to have enough time for yourself. When you get to the last few minutes of the test, it may seem like you won't have enough time left, but if you only have as many questions as you should have left at that point, then you're right on track!

Answer Selection

The best way to pick an answer choice is to eliminate all of those that are wrong, until only one is left and confirm that is the correct answer. Sometimes though, an answer choice may immediately look right. Be careful! Take a second to make sure that the other choices are not equally obvious. Don't make a hasty mistake. There are only two times that you should stop before checking other answers. First is when you are positive that the answer choice you have selected is correct. Second is when time is almost out and you have to make a quick guess!

Check Your Work

Since you will probably not know every term listed and the answer to every question, it is important that you get credit for the ones that you do know. Don't miss any questions through careless mistakes. If at all possible, try to take a second to look back over your answer selection and make sure you've selected the correct answer choice and haven't made a costly careless mistake (such as marking an answer choice that you didn't mean to mark). This quick double check should more than pay for itself in caught mistakes for the time it costs.

Beware of Directly Quoted Answers

Sometimes an answer choice will repeat word for word a portion of the question or reference section. However, beware of such exact duplication – it may be a trap! More than likely, the correct choice will paraphrase or summarize a point, rather than being exactly the same wording.

Slang

Scientific sounding answers are better than slang ones. An answer choice that begins "To compare the outcomes…" is much more likely to be correct than one that begins "Because some people insisted…"

Extreme Statements

Avoid wild answers that throw out highly controversial ideas that are proclaimed as established fact. An answer choice that states the "process should be used in certain situations, if…" is much more likely to be correct than one that states the "process should be discontinued completely." The first is a calm rational statement and doesn't even make a definitive, uncompromising stance, using a hedge word "if" to provide wiggle room, whereas the second choice is a radical idea and far more extreme.

Answer Choice Families

When you have two or more answer choices that are direct opposites or parallels, one of them is usually the correct answer. For instance, if one answer choice states "x increases" and another answer choice states "x decreases" or "y increases," then those two or three answer choices are very similar in construction and fall into the same family of answer choices. A family of answer choices is when two or three answer choices are very similar in construction, and yet often have a directly opposite meaning. Usually the correct answer choice will be in that family of answer choices. The "odd man out" or answer choice that doesn't seem to fit the parallel construction of the other answer choices is more likely to be incorrect.

Special Report: What is Test Anxiety and How to Overcome It?

The very nature of tests caters to some level of anxiety, nervousness or tension, just as we feel for any important event that occurs in our lives. A little bit of anxiety or nervousness can be a good thing. It helps us with motivation, and makes achievement just that much sweeter. However, too much anxiety can be a problem; especially if it hinders our ability to function and perform.

"Test anxiety," is the term that refers to the emotional reactions that some test-takers experience when faced with a test or exam. Having a fear of testing and exams is based upon a rational fear, since the test-taker's performance can shape the course of an academic career. Nevertheless, experiencing excessive fear of examinations will only interfere with the test-takers ability to perform, and his/her chances to be successful.

There are a large variety of causes that can contribute to the development and sensation of test anxiety. These include, but are not limited to lack of performance and worrying about issues surrounding the test.

Lack of Preparation

Lack of preparation can be identified by the following behaviors or situations:

Not scheduling enough time to study, and therefore cramming the night before the test or exam
Managing time poorly, to create the sensation that there is not enough time to do everything

Failing to organize the text information in advance, so that the study material consists of the entire text and not simply the pertinent information

Poor overall studying habits

Worrying, on the other hand, can be related to both the test taker, or many other factors around him/her that will be affected by the results of the test. These include worrying about:

Previous performances on similar exams, or exams in general

How friends and other students are achieving

The negative consequences that will result from a poor grade or failure

There are three primary elements to test anxiety. Physical components, which involve the same typical bodily reactions as those to acute anxiety (to be discussed below). Emotional factors have to do with fear or panic. Mental or cognitive issues concerning attention spans and memory abilities.

Physical Signals

There are many different symptoms of test anxiety, and these are not limited to mental and emotional strain. Frequently there are a range of physical signals that will let a test taker know that he/she is suffering from test anxiety. These bodily changes can include the following:

Perspiring

Sweaty palms

Wet, trembling hands

Nausea

Dry mouth

A knot in the stomach

Headache

Faintness

Muscle tension

Aching shoulders, back and neck

Rapid heart beat

Feeling too hot/cold

To recognize the sensation of test anxiety, a test-taker should monitor him/herself for the following sensations:

The physical distress symptoms as listed above

Emotional sensitivity, expressing emotional feelings such as the need to cry or laugh too much, or a sensation of anger or helplessness

A decreased ability to think, causing the test-taker to blank out or have racing thoughts that are hard to organize or control.

Though most students will feel some level of anxiety when faced with a test or exam, the majority can cope with that anxiety and maintain it at a manageable level. However, those who cannot are faced with a very real and very serious condition, which can and should be controlled for the immeasurable benefit of this sufferer.

Naturally, these sensations lead to negative results for the testing experience. The most common effects of test anxiety have to do with nervousness and mental blocking.

Nervousness

Nervousness can appear in several different levels:

The test-taker's difficulty, or even inability to read and understand the questions on the test

The difficulty or inability to organize thoughts to a coherent form

The difficulty or inability to recall key words and concepts relating to the testing questions (especially essays)

The receipt of poor grades on a test, though the test material was well known by the test taker

Conversely, a person may also experience mental blocking, which involves:

Blanking out on test questions

Only remembering the correct answers to the questions when the test has already finished.

Fortunately for test anxiety sufferers, beating these feelings, to a large degree, has to do with proper preparation. When a test taker has a feeling of preparedness, then anxiety will be dramatically lessened.

The first step to resolving anxiety issues is to distinguish which of the two types of anxiety are being suffered. If the anxiety is a direct result of a lack of preparation, this should be considered a normal reaction, and the anxiety level (as opposed to the test results) shouldn't be anything to worry about. However, if, when adequately prepared, the test-taker still panics, blanks out, or seems to overreact, this is not a fully rational reaction. While this can be considered normal too, there are many ways to combat and overcome these effects.

Remember that anxiety cannot be entirely eliminated, however, there are ways to minimize it, to make the anxiety easier to manage. Preparation is one of the best ways to minimize test anxiety. Therefore the following techniques are wise in order to best fight off any anxiety that may want to build.

To begin with, try to avoid cramming before a test, whenever it is possible. By trying to memorize an entire term's worth of information in one day, you'll be shocking your system, and not giving yourself a very good chance to absorb the information. This is an easy path to anxiety, so for those who suffer from test anxiety, cramming should not even be considered an option.

Instead of cramming, work throughout the semester to combine all of the material which is presented throughout the semester, and work on it gradually as the course goes by, making sure to master the main concepts first, leaving minor details for a week or so before the test.

To study for the upcoming exam, be sure to pose questions that may be on the examination, to gauge the ability to answer them by integrating the ideas from your texts, notes and lectures, as well as any supplementary readings.

If it is truly impossible to cover all of the information that was covered in that particular term, concentrate on the most important portions, that can be covered very well. Learn these concepts as best as possible, so that when the test comes, a goal can be made to use these concepts as presentations of your knowledge.

In addition to study habits, changes in attitude are critical to beating a struggle with test anxiety. In fact, an improvement of the perspective over the entire test-taking experience can actually help a test taker to enjoy studying and therefore improve the overall experience. Be certain not to overemphasize the significance of the grade - know that the result of the test is neither a reflection of self worth, nor is it a measure of intelligence; one grade will not predict a person's future success.

To improve an overall testing outlook, the following steps should be tried:

Keeping in mind that the most reasonable expectation for taking a test is to expect to try to demonstrate as much of what you know as you possibly can. Reminding ourselves that a test is only one test; this is not the only one, and there will be others.

The thought of thinking of oneself in an irrational, all-or-nothing term should be avoided at all costs.

A reward should be designated for after the test, so there's something to look forward to. Whether it be going to a movie, going out to eat, or simply visiting friends, schedule it in advance, and do it no matter what result is expected on the exam.

Test-takers should also keep in mind that the basics are some of the most important things, even beyond anti-anxiety techniques and studying. Never neglect the basic social, emotional and biological needs, in order to try to absorb information. In order to best achieve, these three factors must be held as just as important as the studying itself.

Study Steps

Remember the following important steps for studying:

Maintain healthy nutrition and exercise habits. Continue both your recreational activities and social pass times. These both contribute to your physical and emotional well being.

Be certain to get a good amount of sleep, especially the night before the test, because when you're overtired you are not able to perform to the best of your best ability.

Keep the studying pace to a moderate level by taking breaks when they are needed, and varying the work whenever possible, to keep the mind fresh instead of getting bored.

When enough studying has been done that all the material that can be learned has been learned, and the test taker is prepared for the test, stop studying and do something relaxing such as listening to music, watching a movie, or taking a warm bubble bath.

There are also many other techniques to minimize the uneasiness or apprehension that is experienced along with test anxiety before, during, or even after the examination. In fact, there are a great deal of things that can be done to stop anxiety from interfering with lifestyle and performance. Again, remember that anxiety will not be eliminated entirely, and it shouldn't be. Otherwise that "up" feeling for exams would not exist, and most of us depend on that sensation to perform better than usual. However, this anxiety has to be at a level that is manageable.

Of course, as we have just discussed, being prepared for the exam is half the battle right away. Attending all classes, finding out what knowledge will be expected on the exam, and knowing the exam schedules are easy steps to lowering anxiety. Keeping up with work will remove the need to cram, and efficient study habits will eliminate wasted time. Studying should be done in an ideal location for concentration, so that it is simple to become interested in the material and give it complete attention. A method such as SQ3R (Survey, Question, Read, Recite, Review) is a wonderful key to follow to make sure that the study habits are as effective as possible, especially in the case of learning from a textbook. Flashcards are great techniques for memorization. Learning to take good notes will mean that notes will be full of useful information, so that less sifting will need to be done to seek out what is pertinent for studying. Reviewing notes after class and then again on occasion will keep the information fresh in the mind. From notes that have been taken summary sheets and outlines can be made for simpler reviewing.

A study group can also be a very motivational and helpful place to study, as there will be a sharing of ideas, all of the minds can work together, to make sure that everyone understands, and the studying will be made more interesting because it will be a social occasion.

Basically, though, as long as the test-taker remains organized and self confident, with efficient study habits, less time will need to be spent studying, and higher grades will be achieved.

To become self confident, there are many useful steps. The first of these is "self talk." It has been shown through extensive research, that self-talk for students who suffer from test anxiety, should be well monitored, in order to make sure that it contributes to self confidence as opposed to sinking the student. Frequently the self talk of test-anxious students is negative or self-defeating, thinking that everyone else is smarter and faster, that they always mess up, and that if they don't do well, they'll fail the entire course. It is important to decreasing anxiety that awareness is made of self talk. Try writing any negative self thoughts and then disputing them with a positive statement instead. Begin self-encouragement as though it was a friend speaking. Repeat positive statements to help reprogram the mind to believing in successes instead of failures.

Helpful Techniques

Other extremely helpful techniques include:

Self-visualization of doing well and reaching goals

While aiming for an "A" level of understanding, don't try to "overprotect" by setting your expectations lower. This will only convince the mind to stop studying in order to meet the lower expectations.

Don't make comparisons with the results or habits of other students. These are individual factors, and different things work for different people, causing different results.

Strive to become an expert in learning what works well, and what can be done in order to improve. Consider collecting this data in a journal.

Create rewards for after studying instead of doing things before studying that will only turn into avoidance behaviors.

Make a practice of relaxing - by using methods such as progressive relaxation, self-hypnosis, guided imagery, etc - in order to make relaxation an automatic sensation.

Work on creating a state of relaxed concentration so that concentrating will take on the focus of the mind, so that none will be wasted on worrying.

Take good care of the physical self by eating well and getting enough sleep.

Plan in time for exercise and stick to this plan.

Beyond these techniques, there are other methods to be used before, during and after the test that will help the test-taker perform well in addition to overcoming anxiety.

Before the exam comes the academic preparation. This involves establishing a study schedule and beginning at least one week before the actual date of the test. By doing this, the anxiety of not having enough time to study for the test will be automatically eliminated. Moreover, this will make the studying a much more effective experience, ensuring that the learning will be an easier process. This relieves much undue pressure on the test-taker.

Summary sheets, note cards, and flash cards with the main concepts and examples of these main concepts should be prepared in advance of the actual studying time. A topic should never be eliminated from this process. By omitting a topic because it isn't expected to be on the test is only setting up the test-taker for anxiety should it actually appear on the exam. Utilize the course syllabus for laying out the topics that should be studied. Carefully go over the notes that were made in class, paying special attention to any of the issues that the professor took special care to emphasize while lecturing in class. In the textbooks, use the chapter review, or if possible, the chapter tests, to begin your review.

It may even be possible to ask the instructor what information will be covered on the exam, or what the format of the exam will be (for example, multiple choice, essay, free form, true-false). Additionally, see if it is possible to find out how many questions will be on the test. If a review sheet or sample test has been offered by the professor, make good use of it, above anything else, for the preparation for the test. Another great resource for getting to know the examination is reviewing tests from previous semesters. Use these tests to review, and aim to achieve a 100% score on each of the possible topics. With a few exceptions, the goal that you set for yourself is the highest one that you will reach.

Take all of the questions that were assigned as homework, and rework them to any other possible course material. The more problems reworked, the more skill and confidence will form as a result. When forming the solution to a problem, write out each of the steps. Don't simply do head work. By doing as many steps on paper as possible, much clarification and therefore confidence will be formed. Do this with as many homework problems as possible, before checking the answers. By checking the answer after each problem, a reinforcement will exist, that will not be on the exam. Study situations should be as exam-like as possible, to prime the test-taker's system for the experience. By waiting to check the answers at the end, a psychological advantage will be formed, to decrease the stress factor.

Another fantastic reason for not cramming is the avoidance of confusion in concepts, especially when it comes to mathematics. 8-10 hours of study will become one hundred percent more effective if it is spread out over a week or at least several days, instead of doing it all in one sitting. Recognize that the human brain requires time in order to assimilate new material, so frequent breaks and a span of study time over several days will be much more beneficial.

Additionally, don't study right up until the point of the exam. Studying should stop a minimum of one hour before the exam begins. This allows the brain to rest and put things in their proper order. This will also provide the time to become as relaxed as possible when going into the examination room. The test-taker will also have time to eat well and eat sensibly. Know that the brain needs food as much as the rest of the body. With enough food and enough sleep, as well as a relaxed attitude, the body and the mind are primed for success.

Avoid any anxious classmates who are talking about the exam. These students only spread anxiety, and are not worth sharing the anxious sentimentalities.

Before the test also involves creating a positive attitude, so mental preparation should also be a point of concentration. There are many keys to creating a positive attitude. Should fears become rushing in, make a visualization of taking the exam, doing well, and seeing an A written on the paper. Write out a list of affirmations that will bring a feeling of confidence, such as "I am doing well in my English class," "I studied well and know my material," "I enjoy this class." Even if the affirmations aren't believed at first, it sends a positive message to the subconscious which will result in an alteration of the overall belief system, which is the system that creates reality.

If a sensation of panic begins, work with the fear and imagine the very worst! Work through the entire scenario of not passing the test, failing the entire course, and dropping out of school, followed by not getting a job, and pushing a shopping cart through the dark alley where you'll live. This will place things into perspective! Then, practice deep breathing and create a visualization of the opposite situation - achieving an "A" on the exam, passing the entire course, receiving the degree at a graduation ceremony.

On the day of the test, there are many things to be done to ensure the best results, as well as the most calm outlook. The following stages are suggested in order to maximize test-taking potential:

Begin the examination day with a moderate breakfast, and avoid any coffee or beverages with caffeine if the test taker is prone to jitters. Even people who are used to managing caffeine can feel jittery or light-headed when it is taken on a test day.

Attempt to do something that is relaxing before the examination begins. As last minute cramming clouds the mastering of overall concepts, it is better to use this time to create a calming outlook.

Be certain to arrive at the test location well in advance, in order to provide time to select a location that is away from doors, windows and other distractions, as well as giving enough time to relax before the test begins.

Keep away from anxiety generating classmates who will upset the sensation of stability and relaxation that is being attempted before the exam.

Should the waiting period before the exam begins cause anxiety, create a self-distraction by reading a light magazine or something else that is relaxing and simple.

During the exam itself, read the entire exam from beginning to end, and find out how much time should be allotted to each individual problem. Once writing the exam, should more time be taken for a problem, it should be abandoned, in order to begin another problem. If there is time at the end, the unfinished problem can always be returned to and completed.

Read the instructions very carefully - twice - so that unpleasant surprises won't follow during or after the exam has ended.

When writing the exam, pretend that the situation is actually simply the completion of homework within a library, or at home. This will assist in forming a relaxed atmosphere, and will allow the brain extra focus for the complex thinking function.

Begin the exam with all of the questions with which the most confidence is felt. This will build the confidence level regarding the entire exam and will begin a quality momentum. This will also create encouragement for trying the problems where uncertainty resides.

Going with the "gut instinct" is always the way to go when solving a problem. Second guessing should be avoided at all costs. Have confidence in the ability to do well.

For essay questions, create an outline in advance that will keep the mind organized and make certain that all of the points are remembered. For multiple choice, read every answer, even if the correct one has been spotted - a better one may exist.

Continue at a pace that is reasonable and not rushed, in order to be able to work carefully. Provide enough time to go over the answers at the end, to check for small errors that can be corrected.

Should a feeling of panic begin, breathe deeply, and think of the feeling of the body releasing sand through its pores. Visualize a calm, peaceful place, and include all of the sights, sounds and sensations of this image. Continue the deep breathing, and take a few minutes to continue this with closed eyes. When all is well again, return to the test.

If a "blanking" occurs for a certain question, skip it and move on to the next question. There will be time to return to the other question later. Get everything done that can be done, first, to guarantee all the grades that can be compiled, and to build all of the confidence possible. Then return to the weaker questions to build the marks from there.

Remember, one's own reality can be created, so as long as the belief is there, success will follow. And remember: anxiety can happen later, right now, there's an exam to be written!

After the examination is complete, whether there is a feeling for a good grade or a bad grade, don't dwell on the exam, and be certain to follow through on the reward that was promised...and enjoy it! Don't dwell on any mistakes that have been made, as there is nothing that can be done at this point anyway.

Additionally, don't begin to study for the next test right away. Do something relaxing for a while, and let the mind relax and prepare itself to begin absorbing information again.

From the results of the exam - both the grade and the entire experience, be certain to learn from what has gone on. Perfect studying habits and work some more on confidence in order to make the next examination experience even better than the last one.

Learn to avoid places where openings occurred for laziness, procrastination and day dreaming.

Use the time between this exam and the next one to better learn to relax, even learning to relax on cue, so that any anxiety can be controlled during the next exam. Learn how to relax the body. Slouch in your chair if that helps. Tighten and then relax all of the different muscle groups, one group at a time, beginning with the feet and then working all the way up to the neck and face. This will ultimately relax the muscles more than they were to begin with. Learn how to breathe deeply and comfortably, and focus on this breathing going in and out as a relaxing thought. With every exhale, repeat the word "relax."

As common as test anxiety is, it is very possible to overcome it. Make yourself one of the test-takers who overcome this frustrating hindrance.

Special Report: Additional Bonus Material

Due to our efforts to try to keep this book to a manageable length, we've created a link that will give you access to all of your additional bonus material.

Please visit http://www.mometrix.com/bonus948/pednutrition to access the information.

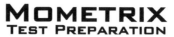

MOMETRIX
TEST PREPARATION
The World's Most Comprehensive Test Preparation Company

Dear Friend,

Thank you for ordering Mometrix products!

We take very seriously that you are entrusting your test preparation needs to us. We have meticulously prepared these materials to ensure we are offering you the most concise, relevant study aid possible. There are many resources available for your exam and we sincerely appreciate you choosing ours to help you attain the highest score within your ability to achieve.

You are about to experience an incredible transformation. Over the next few hours, days, weeks, or months of studying, you will transition from your current level of preparedness to an understanding of the exam content you never thought possible. You now hold in your hands the information you most need to know in order to succeed on your exam. Regardless of whether this is your first time to take the exam or your fifth time, our goal is to give you exactly what you need to maximize your score so you can go where you most want to go and be what you most want to be.

In addition to the products you have ordered from us, we have included a few bonuses that will help in your preparation. Be on the lookout for a special bonus website included in each product that offers additional tips and insights. In response to the test anxiety many people experience, we have also developed a free report to help you overcome this obstacle that you can access by visiting: www.mometrix.com/testanxiety.

From the many families here at Mometrix to yours, we sincerely thank you and wish you the best on your exam and every journey life has in store for you.

If you have any questions or suggestions as to how we can improve our products or service, please contact us at 800-673-8175 or support@mometrix.com.

Sincerely,

Jay Willis
Vice President of Sales
Mometrix Media LLC

P.S. - We would greatly appreciate you recommending our products to your friends and colleagues!